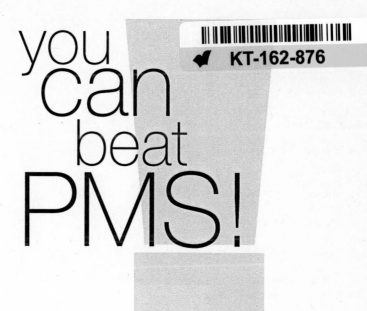

you can beat PMS!

Feel fantastic all month long with this 12-week nutrition and lifestyle plan

COLETTE HARRIS AND THERESA CHEUNG

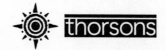

thorsons

Thorsons
An Imprint of HarperCollins*Publishers*
77-85 Fulham Palace Road,
Hammersmith, London W6 8JB

The website address is: www.thorsonselement.com

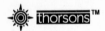

and Thorsons are trademarks
of HarperCollins*Publishers* Ltd

First published by Thorsons 2004

Colette Harris and Theresa Cheung assert the moral right to be
identified as the author of this wor

A catalogue record of this book is
available from the British Library

ISBN 978-0-00-715425-8

NB While the authors of this book have made every effort to ensure that the information
contained in this book is as accurate and up-to-date as possible at the time of publication, medical
and pharmaceutical knowledge is constantly changing and the application of it to particular
circumstances depends on many factors. This book should not be used as an alternative to
specialist medical advice and it is recommended that readers always consult a qualified medical
professional for individual advice before following any new diet or health programme. The author
and publishers cannot be held responsible for any errors and omissions that may be found in the
text, or any actions that may be taken by a reader, as a result of any reliance on the information
contained in the text, which are taken entirely at the reader's own risk.

you
can
beat
PMS!

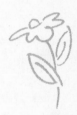

Contents

Foreword

You Can Beat PMS! is a beautifully written and informative account of premenstrual syndrome, the problems it causes and ways to try and deal with the symptoms. Colette Harris and Theresa Cheung are to be congratulated for providing a pragmatic approach to such a highly distressing condition. A novel approach is taken with a day-by-day account of PMS. There is a considerable amount of information on dietary issues and lifestyle changes.

I am certain that this book will be of invaluable support to the many women who experience premenstrual syndrome.

Adam Balen, Consultant Obstetrician and Gynaecologist,
Leeds General Infirmary

Acknowledgements

Colette:
I'd like to thank Chris for his unfailing support, my family, Thorsons, the women who shared their stories with us, the experts who gave us their time and knowledge – most especially Dr Ann Walker – and Theresa, who is full of enthusiasm, energy and commitment, and a real pleasure to work with.

Theresa:
I'd like to thank Ray, Robert and Ruth for their love, support and encouragement, Thorsons, the women we spoke to while researching and writing this book, the experts who shared their wisdom – in particular Dr Ann Walker – and Colette for being such a joy and inspiration to work with.

Introduction

I spend a lot of time and effort trying to outwit the vending machine at work. I love chocolate, full stop – always have done since I was little. So having a vending machine with hot chocolate drinks in it next to a vending machine full of chocolate bars, just a couple of minutes away from my desk, is a nightmare.

I buy bags of fruit at the start of the week and put them on my desk – so that my underlying laziness will make me choose the fruit instead of the two-minute walk.

And generally it works. My mind is busy with other things at work, I eat the snacks at my desk and forget about the vending machine. But there are a couple of days each month when I just can't resist its siren call. I hunger for chocolate to the point where I waste valuable work minutes thinking about it – and finally give in.

On those days I am also dealing with feeling bloated, wearing my softest non-padded bra to minimize the pain of lumpy, tender breasts, and likely to feel tears welling up at the tiniest things, whether it's a moment of high drama on TV, someone pays me a compliment or someone else is a bit offhand. And woe betide the person who pushes me out of the way to get on the bus, or the call centre operator who gets me on the line after I have waited and dialled my way through their company's 10-minute queuing system – because I will be sarcastic and enraged beyond reason.

I always buy ridiculous things I don't need during these two days, too, and get upset about feeling fat and ugly and unfit. And I don't sleep very well, but the upside is the vivid dreams and relentless flow of creative thinking and ideas.

This is my experience of PMS. It's a pattern of emotional and physical symptoms that pops up pretty much regular as clockwork. And as I'm someone who didn't have periods for a while, and had really irregular periods for a longer while than that, due to having a hormonal health condition called PCOS, which one in 10 UK women have – I'll admit to being grateful to have this monthly blip as I first started recovering from PCOS, because it told me my period was on its way.

PCOS is a condition of hormonal imbalance where you feel like you're in permanent PMS state – swollen, irritable, weepy, tender, depressed, angry, desperate for sweet foods (and on top of that you can get any number of symptoms, from excess face and body hair to acne – if that sounds like you, find out more about PCOS in 'Could There Be Another Cause?' on pages 300–1). It was only when I got the PCOS hormonal imbalances sorted out and actually got my regular periods back that I started to experience these other symptoms as part of a cycle – and finally realized I had PMS.

At first – and we're talking six years ago now – I was pleased because I didn't feel like this all the time anymore. It seemed like a relief to have just days of the emotional nightmare. But six years on, with my PCOS under control, I'm thinking wait a minute, PMS is a pain, it leaves me tired and snappy and bloated and uncomfortable two or three days a month. So I started reading up on it – and found out that some women have this going on for weeks. That where I feel weepy and more readily annoyed, some women get so low they feel truly depressed, so angry they feel violent, so foggy-brained that they can't think straight enough to get through their day properly, so bloated and tender they have to have a special larger bra and 'PMS trousers' so their usual waistband doesn't cut into them.

And the worst of it is that many of these women – and maybe you're one of them – don't realize it's within their power to stop feeling like this with some simple, effective changes in what they eat, how they live and how they take care of themselves. Scarily that's because many women with PMS don't even realize they've got it – that's just how they have always felt. And even if it affects their family lives, relationships, work and social lives, they have put up with it.

From my experiences, I can tell you that what I eat, how stressed I am and how well I sleep have a massive effect on how bad I feel in the run up to my period, and how bad I feel during my period. Most months I'm down to two or three days of PMS style symptoms – but some months, when stress and tension leave my period late, it can be seven or eight days. And the thought of other women experiencing this or much worse every month made me feel this book was a book that needed to be written.

I have experienced the incredible power of nutrition, herbs, stress management and exercise in dealing with PCOS, taming hormones with a healthy living approach. So I got together with Theresa and we started digging out research about the same sort of DIY approach to PMS – one of the themes that kept coming through in what we read and from the women we talked to was that PMS makes you feel out of control of your body and out of control of your self. But taking action with self-help strategies – as long as they work! – is a really satisfying way to take that control back.

We were quite surprised to find the amount of research that we did discover. PMS is finally being taken seriously it seems, by the medical community and more members of the general public – good news for women with PMS and the people in their lives who are affected by it. But the fact that lots of research shows various things in your diet and lifestyle can make PMS worse or make it better is one thing – how, when you're already feeling awful, stressed, bloated, emotional out of control and leading a busy life, can you put it all together to make it work in your day-to-day life?

That's where this 12-week plan comes in – because we have translated the information from the experts into a common sense practical plan that will help you transform your health, to feel brighter, more positive, less bloated, less in the grip of mood swings and sugar cravings, and more able to enjoy all the good things life throws at you, as well as coping better with anything stressful that comes your way.

It isn't easy to change your diet and lifestyle – and 12 weeks isn't a miracle overnight cure. But that's because it takes your body a while to heal itself when it has been struggling with a health condition for years. And if you add up the number of days in your life that have been stolen from you due to PMS so far, and think about the number of days in the years to come that will be stolen from you if you don't find a way to deal with it, then 12 weeks starts to seem like an investment worth making. Everything in this plan, from the meals to the exercises, the stress management suggestions and emotional well-being boosters, comes from health experts and other women like you, me and Theresa who have experienced PMS.

We both sincerely hope that you feel better than you could ever have imagined once you have taken the time to follow it through. I for one have felt much more able to sleep, much less bloated and much less likely to cry when someone is nice to me than I have in a long time after following the healthy living guidelines laid out in this book. It's also helped me stay away from the chocolate machine at work – and what a kick that gave me!

Here's hoping you get a kick out of feeling happier and healthier all month long, too.

Colette and Theresa
September 2003

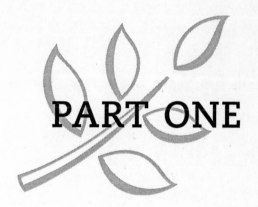

PART ONE

Preparing to Beat PMS

Why You Need to Deal with PMS: The low-down on this condition and its causes

PMS is often joked about, but if you get it you know that feeling this way is anything but a joke: life can become an unhappy, uncomfortable ride.

The worst thing about my PMS is that I feel so out of control. I can't concentrate on work. I overreact to situations at home and I can't relax. My motivation and focus go and I can't seem to handle the simplest task, like deciding what to wear in the morning. I'm an intelligent, capable woman, but PMS takes away my confidence. **Amy, 35**

I don't even need to look at the calendar to know that my period will be arriving in a week or so. I know all the signs. I get furious about the least little thing and get tearful about everything and everyone. Then there are my swollen breasts, puffy stomach and my huge appetite for sweets and chocolate. **Lucy, 29**

I tossed and turned for half the night and woke up tired. I knew I had PMS. The only time I can't sleep is a few days before my period. I dragged myself into work, even though I really wanted to spend the day on the sofa with a box of chocolates, a good book and a purring cat on my lap. **Sophie, 32**

If you don't feel good physically and emotionally in the run-up to your period, this is bound to affect you in all sorts of ways. Studies[1] confirm what you probably already know: PMS can, as Natalie, 41, says, 'screw your life up'.

Research[2] shows that over 90 per cent of women feel that they would be more productive at home and work if they did not have PMS. In her numerous books and studies on PMS, Dr Katharina Dalton of University College Hospital in London, who pioneered research on PMS in the 1950s, shows how the symptoms associated with PMS can and do affect all areas of a woman's life.

PMS isn't just a figment of your imagination. It's unpleasant and uncomfortable. It can make you feel lousy, and can make those you care about feel insecure and uncertain. It can wreak havoc on just about every area of your life: work, relationships, family and friends. That's why you need to deal with it. How can you live your life to the full if you feel ticked off, unhappy and bloated half the time?

What Is PMS?

Dr Raymond Greene and Dr Katharina Dalton first named pre-menstrual syndrome as a medical disorder in a paper published in the *British Medical Journal* in 1953. Dalton describes[3] it as one of the world's oldest and most common diseases caused by hormonal fluctuations that affect the mood, sleep and appetite of a large number of women. The *American Journal of Psychiatry* lists PMS as a physical and psychological disorder that causes symptoms severe enough to 'interfere with some aspects of life, and which appear with a consistent and predictable relationship to menses'.

Put simply, premenstrual syndrome, or PMS, is a mixture of symptoms that affect your physical and emotional health and well-being, for up to two weeks before each menstrual period. These symptoms usually appear about halfway through your cycle and become more intense the week before your period. When your period begins, symptoms are usually reduced or completely disappear.

What Are the Symptoms?

Medical books list more than 150 symptoms associated with PMS. The most common ones include abdominal bloating, water retention, constipation, breast tenderness, fatigue, junk-food binges, clumsiness and mood changes such as irritability, tension, crying spells and anxiety. Some women experience PMS in mild enough forms and it poses no real problem; for others the symptoms can be severe.

You may not have the same set of problems each month, and some months may be definitely worse than others. Your symptoms may also be very different from someone else's. PMS HELP, a national charity in Britain, found in a survey of their members that the average number of symptoms was seven, though some women had as many as thirteen. The seven symptoms included both physical and emotional symptoms, but no two women had the same seven. The variations were endless.

PSYCHOLOGICAL SYMPTOMS ASSOCIATED WITH PMS
- Depression
- Mood swings
- Anger
- Tension
- Inability to cope
- Insecurity
- Low self-esteem
- Fearfulness
- Irrational thoughts
- Jealousy
- Feelings of guilt
- Poor judgement
- Loneliness
- Lethargy

- Clumsiness
- Irritability
- Agitation
- Sleep problems
- Nervousness
- Short temper
- Withdrawal of affection
- Nervous tension
- Forgetfulness
- Periods of confusion and disorientation
- Erratic behaviour
- Crying spells
- Anxiety
- A desire to run away
- Suicidal thoughts

PHYSICAL SYMPTOMS ASSOCIATED WITH PMS

- Menstrual cramps
- Abdominal bloating
- Water retention
- Skin problems
- Headaches
- Backache – especially in lower back
- Breasts enlargement and/or tenderness
- Increased appetite
- Food cravings
- Sugar cravings
- Dizziness
- Acne
- Weight gain
- Lack of co-ordination
- Aches and pains
- Fainting
- Changes in sex drive
- Excessive thirst
- Nausea

- Cramp
- Runny nose
- Sore throat
- Alcohol intolerance
- Piles
- Hives
- Herpes
- Light or noise intolerance
- Restlessness
- Fatigue
- Insomnia
- Candida
- Joint pain
- Weight gain
- Constipation or diarrhoea
- Heart palpitations
- Low blood sugar
- Dizziness
- Allergies
- Fainting
- Asthma
- Eye infections
- Mouth ulcers

PMDD

In a tiny percentage of cases – between 2 and 9 per cent – symptoms are so extreme they become destructive. The most severe form of premenstrual disorder is called premenstrual dysphoric disorder, or PMDD. While PMS is like having thunderstorms for a week or so each month, PMDD is more like an earthquake that can tear up your life for up to two weeks.

PMDD symptoms are similar to deep depression. The difference is that symptoms occur in the days before your period and subside thereafter. Physical symptoms will also accompany the mood changes, and appetite increases often lead to weight gain. To be diagnosed with PMDD, you must experience five or more of the following: anxiety and tension, mood swings, irritability, fatigue, depression, change in appetite, sleep difficulties, feeling overwhelmed and out of control, and physical symptoms such as bloating and breast tenderness. When diagnosing PMDD, physical symptoms are classed together as one symptom as the focus tends to be on the behavioural, psychological and emotional symptoms.

If you suspect you have PMDD, the condition can be managed. This book will help you, but it is vital that you also seek medical help to get the support, advice and treatment you need and deserve.

PMM

PMS can also aggravate other health conditions you may have, such as depression, asthma, allergies and irritable bowel syndrome among others, or make them harder to manage. This is called premenstrual magnification (PMM) and is defined as an underlying health problem you have all month long that worsens 7 to 14 days before the onset of menstruation.

Feeling Helpless

The way you experience PMS may be very different from the way another woman experiences it, but feeling helpless and out of control is a common theme:

> Normally I eat healthily and exercise regularly, but in the week before my period my diet goes out of the window. Why do I do everything I know I shouldn't? **Mary, 26**

> I'm out of control. If anyone does something to annoy me, like cutting in front of me in traffic or slamming a door in my face, I see red.
> **Michelle, 44**

I don't know who I am for half of the month. Nothing makes sense. I love my family but hate them. I enjoy my job but can't be bothered to make an effort. It's like I'm on a seesaw. **Sam, 34**

Fortunately, after you have worked through the 12-week programme in this book you won't feel so powerless and confused anymore. You'll learn that you don't need to feel helpless or out of control when PMS strikes because you can provide yourself with many of the solutions you need with simple changes to your diet and lifestyle.

What Causes PMS?

Although PMS is a recognized medical problem, it is still commonly misdiagnosed and misunderstood by doctors. Perhaps you have read different books and seen various experts give entirely different answers. This is largely because the symptoms and causes vary so much between women. PMS is a puzzle, but one thing is sure: It is linked to your menstrual cycle. Studies[4] show that if a woman is pregnant, or has a hysterectomy, symptoms usually disappear.

Let's take a look at some of the explanations for PMS that you are most likely to hear or read about.

HORMONAL CULPRITS

Studies[5] have shown that an imbalance in levels of progesterone and oestrogen hormone can trigger PMS symptoms. Progesterone is produced in the ovaries along with oestrogen, and while oestrogen can increase energy, progesterone acts as a depressant. For this reason the right level of progesterone and oestrogen create a balance and you feel good – but if the hormonal scales tip out of balance, this may cause PMS.

Too much or too little serotonin may also be a cause according to recent research,[6] as can too much adrenaline and too much androgen.[7] Poor thyroid function[8] has also been linked to PMS.

THE ROLE OF BLOOD SUGAR LEVELS

Problems with glucose tolerance are also thought to be a contributing factor. This theory[9] has been suggested because of symptoms such as food cravings. When high levels of oestrogen occur, more insulin is released into the bloodstream and blood sugar levels dip, causing you to want to eat more. Low blood sugar could explain bingeing on carbohydrates and craving for chocolate during the pre-menstrual phase.

NUTRITIONAL PROBLEMS

Many experts believe that nutritional deficiencies lie at the heart of PMS. Not getting enough of the essential vitamins, minerals and other nutrients can be caused by diet or by outside forces like stress and pollution, when your body uses up more nutrients in order to protect itself.

Studies[10] have linked problems in how the body handles calcium to PMS. Poor diet and deficiency in essential fatty acids, vitamin B6[11] calcium and magnesium[12] have also been associated with PMS in many women. Eating the right kinds of foods can correct the underlying hormonal problems that lie at the root of PMS and tackle specific symptoms, like bloating, depression, anxiety and headaches.

RUNS IN THE FAMILY

Another theory[13] suggests that PMS is an inherited problem. If your mother or another close family member suffered from PMS, you may develop similar problems.

STRESS

If you feel tired or stressed, this may also influence your PMS. Although it probably isn't the only cause, it may play a role in triggering your symptoms or making them worse. We do know that stress affects the functioning of the adrenal glands, which produce a number of hormones that regulate water balance, appetite and mood. One study published in the April 1990 issue of the *Journal of Obstetrics and Gynecology* showed that the use of stress-management techniques resulted in a 58 per cent reduction in symptoms.

Other studies[14] show that stress caused by emotional problems or conflicts can disrupt hormonal balance and trigger symptoms of PMS. According to Dr Christiane Northrup, holistic physician and former president of the American Holistic Medical Association, when women are able to understand and manage their emotions this can help balance their hormones. 'The process of healing our emotional and psychological stress results in biochemical changes in our bodies.'

The PMS Puzzle

We know a lot more about PMS than we did 30 years ago, but the exact cause still remains a puzzle. For every theory above there is one to prove otherwise.

The conclusion many experts come to is that it may not be the hormones themselves or lifestyle factors that trigger PMS symptoms, but a woman's individual response to these hormones or lifestyle factors.[15] So you, and the unique way your body copes with the demands placed on it, are key when it comes to solving the PMS puzzle.

HOW YOU CAN SOLVE IT

Although the exact cause may be hard to pinpoint, it is possible to take what we do know and create a personal course of treatment tailored to your needs. Along with hormonal balance, the effects of your mind, emotions, exercise, diet, relationships, lifestyle, hereditary, and childhood experiences must all be taken into account when treating PMS. The 12-week plan in this book combines the best of conventional and alternative therapy to give you all you need to create your own personal programme for physical, mental and emotional health that can help you solve the riddle of your PMS and rid yourself of it for good.

Who Gets PMS?

Medical research suggests that up to 90 per cent of women experience symptoms of PMS in their menstruating years, and that 40 per cent find that it interferes with their daily life.[16]

THE PMS QUIZ
1 Do you feel anxious or moody a week or so before your period?
2 Do you feel depressed, hopeless, confused or out of control before you are due?
3 Do you have bloating or fluid-retention in the week or so before your period?
4 Do you get headaches or migraines or have difficulty sleeping before your period?
5 Do you get food cravings before you are due?

If you've answered 'yes' to just one of the above questions, you do experience PMS.

PMS can strike in your teens or twenties, but the time when you are most likely to develop PMS is during your thirties. PMS is sometimes called 'the mid-thirties syndrome'. It tends to get worse as you get older, especially after times of hormonal change like stopping the Pill or having a baby. Many women say that over the years symptoms last longer and get more intense. This may be because as we get older our bodies have to work harder to deal with hormonal changes as we take on more responsibilities, leading to stress. The busier you are, the easier it is to let stress, lack of exercise, weight problems and poor diet unsettle your hormones.

You Can Take Control

There is more help for PMS than ever before, and with the 12-week plan outlined here you'll have everything you need for month-long vitality. You don't have to spend your remaining years until menopause feeling like your life is an out-of-control roller-coaster. 'PMS can be recognized, correctly diagnosed and successfully treated,' says PMS expert Dr Katharina Dalton. 'It is a real and treatable condition.'

If you follow the 12-week plan you'll discover that it is possible to feel good all month long. You'll see that the changes you can make transform you from someone who feels like a PMS sufferer to someone who has reclaimed her life and become her real self again. The plan puts you in control of your own health – a powerful experience that will carry over into other areas of your life. So don't suffer any longer or put your life on hold for up to 14 days every month. Use the 12-week plan and start living life to the full.

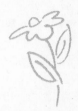

How and Why the 12-week Plan Works

PMS can rob you of the two most precious gifts that you have – your health and your peace of mind. Over the next 12 weeks you can recover these lost gems and improve your health, your mood and your well-being. It will take patience and persistence, so this chapter will explain why the plan requires you to make changes.

How the Plan Works

Drawing on personal experiences and the latest research from conventional and alternative medicine, the 12-week plan is a combination of self-care activities, lifestyle changes, dietary supplements and coping strategies whose purpose is to beat PMS. All you need to do is read the advice for each week and then gently incorporate the changes and recommendations into your life, week by week, for a 12-week period. We have broken all the exercises, information and recommendations down into small, bite-sized pieces so you can easily digest and integrate them into your life. There is nothing complicated or difficult here, and you'll be surprised how easy the plan is to use and work into your life. Follow the weekly guidelines and by the end of the 12 weeks you will notice a significant reduction in your symptoms and an improved sense of well-being.

Setting the Scene

As you work through the plan you'll notice that every week we explore four key areas:

1 Nutrition
2 Exercise
3 Emotional well-being
4 Vitality boosters

Research has shown that these are the areas that can help you beat PMS on your own or with the help of any medication from your doctor. (For PMS medications, see Appendix 1.) In the next few pages we'll explain why these four areas are so effective in the treatment of PMS. There's a lot of information to take in, but don't worry – we are just setting the scene. You aren't being asked to make *all* the changes suggested straight away. To be effective, lifestyle changes need to be incorporated gradually into your life – and we'll give advice about how you can do this over the next 12 weeks. The important thing right now is to focus on the *why*, not the *how*. Being informed and knowing why you are being asked to do something will be a great incentive when you work through the plan over the next 12 weeks.

Good Nutrition

Food is like fuel. It gives your body the energy it needs to function well. If you don't make sure that the fuel you pump into your body is of the right quality or quantity, you won't feel as healthy as you should. What you eat is the foundation for good health – and this is especially true if you have PMS, because what, when and how much you eat *directly* affects the severity of your symptoms.

There is general agreement among experts that the first line of treatment for PMS should be dietary.[1] Links have been found between the foods you eat and symptoms of PMS, and changing the way you eat can ease your symptoms.[2] PMS is associated not only with hormonal imbalance but also with blood sugar fluctuations and deficiencies of certain nutrients. It is possible for you to ease or erase many PMS symptoms by making informed food choices.

> *The run-up to my period was always an emotional time. I'd feel so low and only sweet food and caffeine could give me an immediate emotional lift. But by the time I was 30 I was so addicted to caffeine that I began to notice how it was making things much worse. I made the decision to cut down for a month to see if my PMS got better. It did. This was the wake-up call I needed. I finally realized just how much of an effect my diet had on how I felt. I did some reading on healthy eating and started to cut down my sugar and salt intake. Problems with bloating and headaches disappeared. It was amazing. And after a few more weeks of healthy eating, I didn't feel so tired and emotional either.* **Elizabeth, 38**

So how do you eat right for PMS? Fortunately, the dietary guidelines for managing PMS are in sync with the fundamental nutritional requirements for a healthy body and mind. There are seven basic principles of healthy eating outlined below, together with the reasons why eating well can help banish your monthly blues.

As you work through the 12-week plan we'll show you how you can incorporate these seven principles into your life. We'll also refer back to this section in the weeks ahead and discuss the key strategies, supplements and specific dietary tips that can make all the difference to how you feel.

The Seven Principles of Healthy Eating

1) DRINK MORE WATER

Headaches, fatigue, dizziness and stomach upsets are all symptoms of PMS, right? Yes they are, but they could also be symptoms of dehydration.

Water is an essential and often forgotten nutrient. Without it we could not last more than a few days. Our bodies are made up of two-thirds water, and water intake and distribution is vital for hormonal function. You need to drink lots of water – about 8 large glasses a day – to keep your hormonal systems working at their best. Water also keeps your skin healthy and your eyes sparkling. It delivers nutrients to your organs and helps the body eliminate waste and toxins by making the fibre in your food swell and perform its function, and without it, you can feel dizzy, tired and bloated – not helpful when you are dealing with PMS!

2) EAT FIVE PORTIONS OF FRUIT AND VEGETABLES A DAY

A recent study by the National Health Survey for England showed that only one in four people eat enough fruit and vegetables to help protect them from health problems. Young people eat even less – just one in five, claims the study. (We'll take a look at what makes up a 'portion' on pages 166–7.)

If you have PMS, vegetables and most fruits are essential. Not only do the vitamins, minerals and other nutrients they contain help balance fluctuating hormone levels and ease PMS, they can keep your bones strong, boost your immune system, calm the nervous system, ease depression, aid digestion and ease bloating because of their fibre content.

Research[3] has shown that certain vitamin and mineral deficiencies, in particular calcium and magnesium, may either cause PMS or make it worse. We'll explore this in more detail over the next few weeks, but for now just bear in mind that vegetables and fruits are rich in vitamins, minerals and other nutrients that research has shown can ease many premenstrual symptoms. For example, vitamin B6 – found in spinach, lentils and bananas – can ease depression, irritability, mood swings, breast tenderness, fatigue, acne and water retention. Vitamin C – found in Brussels sprouts, green leafy vegetables and citrus fruits – can help fight fatigue, aches and pains, sugar cravings, water retention and breast tenderness. Vitamin E – found in sweet potatoes, asparagus and green beans – can ease breast tenderness, depression, insomnia and fatigue. Calcium – found in spinach and green leafy vegetables – can ease water retention, food cravings, mood swings and headaches. Magnesium – found in beans, peas and green leafy vegetables – can ease water retention, headaches, mood swings and fatigue.

So, it's for these reasons that in the next 12 weeks you'll be eating lots of fruit and veg.

3) BALANCE BLOOD SUGAR

Irritability, mood swings, forgetfulness, anxiety, confusion, problems with concentration, feeling tearful, food cravings, fatigue and headaches are all symptoms of PMS. They are also symptoms of fluctuating blood sugar levels. Many experts believe that balancing blood sugar levels is the best treatment for PMS.[4] It is thought that changes in your body chemistry in the week before your period, when your body is gearing up for a possible pregnancy, make your body much more sensitive to insulin, the hormone that helps stabilize glucose levels in your blood. Many women end up with lower-than-usual levels of blood glucose, and that's why you feel fed up, irritable and moody. It's also why you get food cravings – usually for sweet foods.

If blood sugar levels aren't balanced this will also trigger the production of adrenaline, which not only increase feelings of stress but also blocks the uptake of progesterone in your body, triggering symptoms of PMS. If blood sugar levels are stable, however, progesterone is released and symptoms are not triggered. The blood sugar level theory explains why women with PMS may have similar amounts of progesterone and oestrogen to women without. Their bodies release enough progesterone, but just can't make use of it because of fluctuating blood sugar levels.

In the 12-week plan, you'll be eating to keep blood sugar steady in three main ways:

i) Eating Regular Healthy Snacks
Eating a wide variety of nutrient-rich foods in five or six meals a day is thought to be one of the best ways to combat PMS irritability, aggression, fatigue, dizziness, clumsiness and headaches. Why? Because all these symptoms are associated with low blood sugar which often occurs in the premenstrual phase.
You'll notice that all the sample daily menus in our plan revolve around three meals and two or three snacks a day: a decent breakfast, a mid-morning snack, followed by lunch, a mid-afternoon snack and supper. That way you'll never get too hungry and your blood sugar levels remain stable. It isn't a good idea to skip meals or fast. The aim is to keep blood sugar stable with a regular supply of nutrient-rich food.

ii) Eating Protein with Each Meal
Protein helps balance your blood sugar, preventing the dips and highs in blood sugar that can bring about many PMS symptoms. Protein also gives your body an even supply of the amino acids it needs to build and repair cells and manufacture hormones and brain chemicals. Since your body can't store protein, as it does carbohydrates and fat, you need a constant supply. That's why you need to eat small portions of good-quality protein with every meal.

Eating too much protein means that you have less room for nutrient-rich foods that can also help balance blood sugar, so it isn't wise to overload on protein. A sensible balance is to eat two portions of carbohydrates (see below) to every one portion of protein. You'll find that incorporating protein in your meals is actually quite simple: for breakfast you might have toast with peanut butter, or cereal with milk; for lunch you might have chili with beans, or whole-wheat pita bread with hummus; for dinner you could have rice with beans, or wholemeal pasta with chicken.

iii) Choosing the Right Carbs
There are two kinds of carbohydrates. Complex carbohydrates take longer to convert to glucose, giving you sustained energy and hormone balance. Potatoes, brown pasta, vegetables, dried fruits and wholemeal breads are typical sources of complex carbohydrates. Simple sugars, on the other hand – as found in refined foods, sweets, cakes, biscuits, and some fruits – tend to raise blood sugar too quickly. That's why you need to change the type of carbohydrates you eat rather than cutting them out altogether.

Experts differ, but in general it is thought that a healthy diet should consist of around 40 to 50 per cent carbohydrates. In addition to the carbohydrate in fruit and vegetables, which count towards your daily 50 per cent, the rest of your intake should come from complex, low GI (glycaemic index) carbs.

THE GLYCAEMIC INDEX
The Glycaemic Index is used as a guideline for people with hypoglycaemia or diabetes. Carbohydrate foods are classified into three main groups according to how fast they are turned into blood sugar by your body. The higher a food appears on the glycaemic index, the faster it raises blood sugar. The lower the GI, the more slowly the food will convert into blood sugar, promoting hormonal balance.

Glycaemic Index of Some Foods

SUGARS		VEGETABLES	
Glucose	100	Carrot, raw	31
Honey	75	Carrot, cooked	36
Sucrose	60	Potato, baked	98
Fructose	20	Potato, boiled	70

FRUITS	
Apples	39
Bananas	62
Oranges	40
Orange juice	46
Raisins	64

A quick way to work out the GI of a particular food without resorting to charts is to think about how refined it is. If it is highly refined, i.e., lots of sugar, salt, additives and preservatives, it is going to make symptoms of PMS worse. The less refined carbs – for example those found in brown rice, whole grains and vegetables – are going to lower blood sugar. Choose foods that are as close as possible to their raw or natural state, and base your diet on foods that are rich in fibre.

The Glycaemic Index is helpful if you have PMS, but it should not be the only dietary guideline on which to base your food choices. When a food has both carbohydrate and protein in it, for example lentils, this lowers the GI. So when eating carbohydrates it is important to combine them with a little protein. For example, a baked potato has a high GI, but if you eat it with some tuna or low-fat cottage cheese it has a stabilizing effect on blood sugar.

4) EAT A HIGH-FIBRE DIET
Fibre, like protein, is important for PMS because it slows down the release of blood sugar, thus helping maintain blood-sugar balance.

It also keeps your digestion healthy, allowing waste to pass through at a steady rate, ensuring less bloating and preventing the build-up of hormones and toxins being reabsorbed into the bloodstream.

In the next 12 weeks you'll aim to eat 30 to 50 g of fibre daily. This isn't a great amount but you still need to drink plenty of fluids to ensure it passes through your digestive system. You can get your fibre in wholegrain foods, nuts, seeds, fruits and vegetables. As a rough guide, an apple has around 2 g of fibre and an orange 3 g. Eat your five portions of fruit and vegetables a day and you are halfway there.

5) MAKE SURE YOU GET ENOUGH ESSENTIAL FATTY ACIDS (EFAs)

If you are eating too little fat or too much of the wrong kind of fat, you won't be getting enough essential fats (EFA) and this could trigger symptoms of PMS.

Your body needs essential fats to regulate hormone function. If you are eating enough essential fatty acids in your diet, not only will your skin, hair and nails feel healthy and strong, but symptoms will also ease. This is because EFAs satisfy your hunger, slow down the entry of carbohydrates and keep blood sugar levels lower. Without the right amount of EFAs your body can't manufacture many important substances, including ovarian hormones.

As a guideline, around 20 to 25 per cent of your diet should come from good fat, such as omega 3 and 6 fatty acids found in nuts, seeds, olive oil and oily fish (mackerel, salmon, herrings and sardines). Aim to eat fish at least twice a week, and nuts and seeds (flax, sunflower, pumpkin, sesame, hemp, almonds, cashews, walnuts) daily, maybe as a snack between meals. You can take linseed (flax) oil by the tablespoon or in salad dressings, add hempseed oil to smoothies, or use sesame oil with stir-fries.

Unlike saturated animal fats or the transfatty fats found in many commercial foods, which have no nutritional function, essential fats help to reduce swelling and inflammation of the body – if you get swollen, tender breasts and abdomen due to PMS, they are real power foods. And healthy skin that's spot-free is encouraged by EFAs, so they really are the good guys.

6) STOCK UP ON PHYTONUTRIENTS

Phytonutrients, or phytochemicals, are health-supporting substances found in plants, offering natural protection against all kinds of diseases and reducing the risk of diabetes, heart disease and memory loss. Certain phytonutrients also have a balancing effect on oestrogen levels, increasing them when they are low and decreasing them when they are too high.[5] As such they can be an effective way to treat hormonal imbalance and symptoms of PMS. These nutrients are called phytoestrogens and they occur especially in soya, flax seeds, wheat, rice, oats, barley, carrots, potatoes, apples, cherries, plums, parsley and in herbs such as sage leaf, hops and liquorice. Vegetable oils, including safflower, wheat germ, corn linseed (flaxseed) , peanut, olive, soya and coconut oils may also be high in phtyoestrogens.

7) GET SPICY

If you have problems with PMS water retention, bloating, weight gain or breast swelling, this could be the result of too much salt in your diet. The more you eat the more your body holds on to water in your tissues to avoid dehydration. So if you tend to retain water, the more salt (sodium) you eat, the worse your problem gets. Fluid retention can raise blood pressure as well.

You can't avoid salt altogether, but you can take steps to reduce your sodium intake. Instead of salt, try using herbs, spices, lemon juice, wine or ginger to flavour your food. Have fun experimenting with spices and alternatives until you find those that you like best. Check the salt content of foods you eat. There are hidden salts in most of the foods we buy and eat today, especially ones that have chemicals, additives and preservatives in them. Some foods claim to be 'reduced salt' or 'low salt', but this can be confusing as most manufacturers are talking about sodium rather than salt. To find out how much salt there is in the food, you multiply the sodium content by 2.5. Aim for less than 5 g a day. In time you will get used to a less salty diet and start to really taste food again free from the overpowering taste of salt.

MAKING SURE YOUR PMS DIET IS A SUCCESS

The seven principles of healthy eating outlined above will help to balance your blood sugar levels and ease your symptoms. Over the next 12 weeks we are going to give you recipes, advice and suggestions to help you incorporate these principles into your life. Remember, though, that changing the way you eat takes time. Make small changes and as each week passes you will start to notice gradual improvements in your symptoms and the way you look and feel.

Try not to set yourself up for failure and remember the 80/20 rule. The occasional treat doesn't mean you have failed. It is the excesses that can trigger symptoms. Eat healthily for most (80 per cent) of the time but allow yourself the occasional indulgence. You're not going to have to give up all your favourite foods, you just need to eat them in moderation. No food is banned completely in the PMS diet. But over time as you make small gradual improvements, the dramatic changes in how you feel will spur you on to make changes that you never dreamed possible.

I didn't think I had any willpower but it took me less than a month to cut down on refined sugar in my diet. Once I made the decision everything fell into place. I can't believe I used to heap three teaspoons of sugar in my teacup or on my cereal in the morning. I just wouldn't be able to do that now. I've started to taste my food for the first time in years, and there's no looking back. **Monica, 37**

I really didn't think I could stick to a healthy eating plan. I loved coffee, chocolate, wine and junk food. I started by making gradual changes and immediately the headaches stopped. Spurred on by the improvement I was encouraged to make other changes. It took about four months to completely change my diet and for my symptoms to disappear. **Mary, 40**

The most effective way to treat PMS isn't through medication or hormone therapy but through a balancing diet that can regulate your hormones and blood sugar levels. You may even find that what you thought was a symptom of PMS disappears when you start eating a balanced diet. Imbalances of blood sugar or stress hormones often trigger symptoms that are indistinguishable from PMS. When you start to eat a better diet or learn to manage stress effectively, you could be miraculously cured of PMS. According to Doctor Marion Stewart from the Women's Nutritional Advisory Service, PMS symptoms vanish in 90 per cent of women within three to four months of making positive changes to their diet, exercising regularly and finding effective ways to manage stress.

The seven principles of healthy eating all work towards the same goal – balancing blood sugar levels, improving your health and easing PMS symptoms. Remember, when it comes to PMS the importance of the food you eat can't be stressed enough. A healthy diet is the best place to start. That's why your quest to beat PMS begins when we help you plan a week of healthy menus.

PMS-busting Exercise

Regular exercise[6] in combination with a healthy diet is essential for women with PMS. Recent research confirms that regular, moderate exercise evokes hormonal responses from the body. Women who[7] engage in moderate aerobic exercise at least three times a week have fewer symptoms than women who don't exercise. In fact, exercise is one of the most effective, healthy and natural ways to combat PMS. It can help with just about every symptom of PMS.

Exercise is wonderful. It boosts my mood and cleans out my body at the same time. It's like putting in new batteries when the old ones have run out. I have no doubt that exercise has a positive effect on my PMS. I'm living proof. I was fairly active at school and college, but then I got a desk-bound job and within a year I was suffering from terrible PMS. Then I was asked to join the office sports team. As well as matches we'd get together twice a week to practice. After three or four months of regular exercise, my PMS disappeared. **Nina, 26**

The American Diabetic Association lists the health benefits of exercise, and many of them are particularly important for women with PMS.
Exercise lowers your blood sugar levels by burning it as fuel. The fitter you are, the lower your body fat and the better your insulin and glucose control.

Steady exercise for more than 20 minutes allows your muscles to store more glucose, lowering your blood sugar levels even after you have stopped exercising.

Exercise can also help with symptoms such as water retention, headaches and depression. This is because when you exercise you supply your tissues with lots of oxygen, which can help eliminate waste that could trigger headaches and water retention. And when you exercise you release hormones called *endorphins*, which help you feel happier and more positive. These endorphins can help ease irritability, mood swings and depression. It has been suggested that women with PMS may have only 20 to 50 per cent of the amount of endorphins circulating as compared to a woman without. Exercise is also a great stress-reliever – and don't we need that when PMS strikes! Exerting yourself physically gives your body an opportunity to release pent-up tensions and anxiety. And finally, it is thought that moderate exercise can suppress the overproduction of hormones and help keep hormones in balance.

For maximum benefits, experts recommend at least 20 minutes of exercise (preferably aerobic) at least three times a week, and every day in the premenstrual phase. So that's why the plan has you walking right from the start!

Emotional Well-being

Stress predisposes us to PMS. When you are under stress, the adrenal glands release hormones that have a blocking effect on progesterone. Stress also increases the body's needs for certain nutrients including vitamin C. And you can't absorb iron effectively from your diet when you are stressed – so stress can contribute to an iron deficiency. Stress may not be the cause of PMS, but it plays a big part in triggering and worsening symptoms.

> It wasn't until my second baby, Jane, was born that PMS got really bad. I was coping OK until then. A few days before my period I'd feel tearful and overwhelmed, but it would soon pass. My first baby, Joseph, was a demanding baby but I had no idea how much harder things would get when I had not one but two demanding kids under five to care for. There were days when I wouldn't even be able to get out of the house, my PMS was so bad. Thank goodness I never lost it with the kids, but I did get very depressed and overweight. It was a huge relief when my mum moved in and I got help with childcare. My PMS hasn't been so bad since. **Sarah, 35**

It's often the small stuff that gets us worked up – missing a train, kids late for school – and it is important if you have PMS to save your stress hormones for real emergencies. That means rethinking how we respond to setbacks and problems and learning ways to put them into perspective. Many studies[8] have shown how successful stress-management techniques have been in managing premenstrual syndrome. And we guarantee that if you can reduce the amount of stress in your life, your symptoms of PMS will also be reduced.

The emotional well-being section of the 12-week plan will help you tackle stress and smooth out mood swings so you aren't a hostage to PMS anymore.

Vitality Boosters

PMS can leave you feeling drained, low, sapped of your spark and desire to enjoy life. Improving your lifestyle – what you eat, how much you exercise, how much you sleep and relax and your relationship with yourself and other people – is guaranteed to add the zest back in! Improving your lifestyle is important for three reasons if you have PMS:

1 Scientists continue to explore how negative states such as stress, anger and fatigue affect the development of PMS. Their research shows that positive states, such as a sense of peacefulness, a sense of humour, high energy levels and an optimistic outlook help fight the effects of PMS.
2 Many doctors believe that the single most important thing in treating PMS is a healthy lifestyle. Simple changes such as getting enough sleep, taking time for you, or eating more fruits and vegetables have worked better than medicine in many cases.
3 When you make lifestyle changes such as ensuring you get quality sleep you are taking control of your life, which is an important step in fighting PMS. Making changes that are positive will give you a feeling of empowerment, which is a valuable life skill, not just a way to beat PMS.

Over the next 12 weeks we'll show you how lifestyle changes that build your self-esteem and raise your energy levels – like taking supplements, sleeping well, lifting your mood, and self-esteem building exercises and DIY exercises like massage or aromatherapy baths – can help you beat PMS. Each week you'll get the chance to focus on one of them to boost your quality of life.

Now that we have set the scene, and explained the theory behind the plan and how it is structured around four key areas – diet, exercise, stress reduction and energy boosting – let's explain *why* it works.

Why the Plan Works

Having PMS is bad enough, but the constant feeling of being below-par can have added effects for your mood and energy levels, so you need to tackle those, too. That's why in addition to addressing any PMS symptoms, the plan will also improve your general health and sense of well-being so that you can keep going all month long at your very best.

In 2002 the first study on well-being revealed that people with a good sense of well-being take greater responsibility for their health, visit the doctor less, and enjoy a better quality of life. Based on extensive academic and expert thinking from the Henley Centre, the Boots study identified 15 factors that make up over two-thirds of our well-being. At the centre of these factors are the 'big five' which remain 'constant' throughout our lives. Although health was one of these, it was outweighed by:

    having a sense of control over life and the direction it takes
    an optimistic outlook
    feeling confident
    feeling valued by others.

What you'll find as you work through the 12-week programme is that you become the one who is in charge of your PMS, health and well-being. That's why the plan works. Using the latest research, it will help you target symptoms of PMS individually, get your diet and exercise levels back on track, manage stress, get support from others if you need it, improve your mood and boost your energy. The guidelines for managing PMS are in sync with all the requirements for well-being, so the plan not only helps you to beat PMS but helps you to look and feel great about yourself and your life.

Imagine just 12 weeks from now, having energy, feeling confident and no longer at the mercy of your symptoms. Research shows that diet, exercise, stress management and a positive attitude can all help enormously with recovery, but perhaps the biggest factor is your ability to take control of your health. It doesn't matter what age you are, how unhealthy your diet or how fit or unfit you are. No matter who you are, the 12-week plan will help you take charge of your health and beat PMS for good.

WHY 12 WEEKS?

Unfortunately there are no quick fixes for PMS. The changes recommended in the plan won't cure PMS overnight. You need to work with us for a 12-week period. It is important that you commit yourself to the 12-week plan so you really get the benefits. Experts[10] agree that 12 weeks, or around three months, is the recommended amount of time for dietary changes to take effect and nutritional supplements and herbs to work their magic. Think about it – your body and mind need time to adjust to the changes. Old habits die hard. You may start feeling better three to four weeks into the programme, but typically you will need at least two menstrual cycles to start to feel the full benefits.

Twelve weeks is also about the amount of time you will need to integrate positive lifestyle changes into your life. According to psychologists – and research backs this up – it takes at least three months to replace dietary and lifestyle habits that aren't doing you any good with healthier ones. So don't get disillusioned if the first month is a bit tough as your body and mind adjust. Remind yourself that if you want to feel better, you have to persist.

Working in Partnership with Your Doctor

The first choice of treatment for PMS is self-help, and you may find that the 12-week plan is all you need to beat PMS – but you may also decide to take some course of medicine, treatment or therapy to manage your symptoms. The guidelines set out in the 12-week plan are the essential foundation for any kind of medication you decide to take. The plan works in conjunction with every medication for PMS, from the Pill (if you are taking the Pill see the guidelines in Part Three: Fine-tuning Your Plan) to oestrogen patches, progesterone creams and alternative therapies.

In her extensive research on treatments for PMS, Dr Katharina Dalton stresses that whatever medication you take 'dietary and lifestyle change is the first step in relief of PMS symptoms'. Basics like a good diet mean that any medication you use works much better. For example, studies on Evening Primrose Oil,[11] which is often used as a treatment for PMS, shows that it is most effective in women who are also eating a healthy diet and taking multivitamins. Alone it is no more effective than a placebo.

Eating healthily and exercising regularly are important for everyone, but if you suffer from PMS they are an essential part of feeling healthy and relieving symptoms. You may find that your doctor discusses healthy lifestyle changes that you can make.

> I suffered with PMS for nine years before my GP referred me to the Women's Nutritional Advisory Service. They gave me a personal plan of changes in my diet, exercise and supplements. After a month my symptoms began to improve. A few more months went by and I start to feel really good. I've got lots more energy, my stomach doesn't get bloated any more and I've stopped feeling so irritable. **Maria, 32**

Dr Ann Walker, a medical herbalist and research scientist based at the University of Reading's High Sinclair Unit of Human Nutrition, who has researched PMS for many years, explains that many herbalists and complementary therapists will suggest beneficial changes to diet and lifestyle as the basis for treating PMS. She stresses that in order for any kind of treatment to achieve results these changes have to be made first. 'Supplements and treatments are what their name suggests, supplemental or extra. They are not a substitute of a healthy diet and lifestyle. There is no point in any kind of medication or therapy coming in to suppress symptoms that are caused by junk food and lack of exercise. It is important to get the diet and lifestyle healthy first and then treat the remaining symptoms with medication or supplements. Any treatments you might need will work far more efficiently when your body is getting optimum nutrition and your lifestyle is healthy.'

If you are on or thinking about any kind of medication for PMS, think of the guidelines in the 12-week plan as the foundation of your treatment.

Freedom from PMS

I've made quite a few changes to my diet and lifestyle over the past few months. I made the changes a little at a time and now they are second nature to me. It's easy to do when the benefits are so great. The biggest change is that now I wake up happy most of the time and I really enjoy things. Then everything was a struggle and I had no patience. The slightest thing would set me off and I would become this person I didn't recognize. It makes me shiver to remember. I've finally managed to sort my PMS out. I've finally discovered what it is like not to have a life controlled by PMS. It feels wonderful. **Tracy, 31**

Having PMS presents you with an opportunity for growth. PMS is a real and complex medical disorder that can be treated, and once you realize this you have the motivation you need to examine your lifestyle. You can approach the 12-week plan as a great way to turn your life around, be free and clear of PMS for ever and feel happy and healthy all month long.

Getting to Know Your Own PMS: Work out now exactly what you want to beat

If you were to describe some PMS symptoms to a friend or a colleague – from feeling tired and irritable, to having sugar cravings, feeling helpless and overwhelmed to breaking out in spots – they'd probably say 'that sounds just like me.' Everyone feels tired, moody, weepy, anxious, headachy, spotty and chocolate-mad sometimes, whether through stress, like money worries, lack of sleep, pressure at work or a thousand other reasons. But before you set out to beat PMS you need to know what you're beating in your own personal case. And that means getting to know your own cycle and symptoms. If you suspect you have PMS, there are two ways that can help you diagnose and treat it. We call these 'recognizing' and 'recording'.

Recognizing

The best way to diagnose PMS with accuracy is to recognize what your symptoms are and when they occur. Earlier we mentioned the huge number of PMS-related symptoms. Professor Guy Abraham, formerly President of Obstetrics and Gynecology at the University of California and Patron of the Women's Nutrition Advisory Service, believes that these symptoms typically fall into four types of PMS sufferers:

1 Type A – experiencing anxiety, irritability and tension
2 Type B – experiencing bloating, swelling and weight gain
3 Type C – experiencing craving for sweets and stodgy foods followed
   by fatigue and headaches
4 Type D – experiencing depression and confusion.[1]

You may find that your symptoms all belong to one type, but it's more likely that you also experience symptoms from more than one group. Whatever your symptoms, the main thing is to recognize them. Once you have done that you can then start to notice if there is a pattern; because *when* they occur is actually more important than what they are.

Recording

Record your symptoms through a typical month. This way you can find out if there is a relationship between your symptoms and your menstrual cycle. If it is PMS, symptoms will cluster in the two weeks before your period starts. (In some cases they may spread into the postmenstrual days too, so that you have only a week or so without symptoms.) If it isn't PMS, symptoms will appear at other times in the month.

We'll show you how to chart your symptoms below, right after we take a closer look at the menstrual cycle.

Menstrual Cycle Summary

The word 'menstruation' comes from *menses*, the Latin word for 'month', and the typical length of a bleed is five to seven days. Your menstrual cycles are never absolutely regular. Using an average length of time, a cycle lasts 28 days, although any cycle from 23 to 35 days is typical. Your cycle begins on the first day of your period. Ovulation occurs between 10 and 14 days before your next period starts. Everyone is unique, though, so bear in mind that the outline below is only a rough guide to what typically happens. You may have a shorter or a longer cycle, or your cycle may be different each month.

You may also not ovulate every month. Some women are aware when they ovulate – they experience mild to sharp pain in their ovaries (just above the pubic bone) and cervical mucus changes (mucus resembles egg white and it is clear and stretchy), but you can have a period without ovulating. When ovulation does not take place the hormone progesterone is not produced.

TIME OF THE MONTH
The hormones that affect your cycle surge, peak and plummet over an average of 28 days. Your cycle is controlled by a complex interaction between oestrogen and progesterone, the pituitary gland and the ovaries. Here's a brief guide to help you through the month.

Days 1-8
Your cycle begins on the day your period starts. Production of the hormone progesterone has fallen so low that your brain (hypothalamus) tells your pituitary gland to release *follicle-stimulating hormone* (FSH) to begin a new cycle.
Around Day 4, production of FSH increases and this triggers the growth of follicles or sacs on the ovary. For the next two weeks these follicles grow and mature, so the first half of your menstrual cycle is called the *follicular phase*. While all this is happening, production of *oestrogen*[2] coming from the ovaries starts to rise and cause the lining of your womb (uterus) to increase. Rising oestrogen means skin starts to improve because oestrogen plays a part in its hydration.

Days 9-16
Oestrogen levels rise and then peak at ovulation, which typically occurs at Day 14. The pituitary slows production of FSH and

releases luteinizing hormone (LH), which causes ovulation: a mature egg (or sometimes more than one egg) is released from the follicle and enters the fallopian tube. Around this time, fertile alkaline mucus is produced in the cervix to produce the right conditions for sperm to travel towards the fallopian tube and possibly fertilize the egg. Because the oestrogen—progesterone balance is changing, skin may get greasy and spotty.

To replace lost iron during your period it's important to eat plenty of green, leafy vegetables and fresh fruit, veg, fish, nuts and seeds packed with essential fatty acids during and after ovulation. It's also a good idea to keep exercising on a regular basis, as oestrogen helps the body store fat and levels of fat-inducing oestrogen are high at the moment.

Days 17-28

The empty follicle left behind is called the *corpus luteum*, and this starts to produce *progesterone*. The second half of your menstrual cycle, called the *luteal phase*, has begun. If a sperm fertilizes the egg, progesterone causes glands in your womb to produce embryo-nourishing substances. If the egg is not fertilized, the production of oestrogen and progesterone start to decrease over the next 10 to 14 days. Lack of *progesterone* causes the uterine lining to shed. We are back to the first day of your menstrual cycle.

WRITE IT DOWN

You don't need to wait until you are symptom-free to start charting your symptoms. Starting today get into the habit of writing down any symptoms – such as headache, bloating, fatigue – and how you feel: happy, sad, weepy, irritable, depressed and so on. Record even the smallest upsets or arguments you have had, and why they happened: 'Saw red when guy cut in front of me in traffic,' 'Furious with children for not eating supper,' and so on.

Just give it a little effort – maybe write it before you go to bed every night or first thing in the morning. Don't just write the negative stuff ('a night mare day. Stomach huge, breasts sore, chocolate consumption hideous') write the positive stuff down, too ('Felt on top of the world today'). This will help put things in perspective for you. You can make your chart elaborate, but you can also keep it simple by using the charts we have provided in the back of the book.

Tracking and recording your symptoms is about much more than simply writing down how you feel, however. It is about self-awareness and can help you become more attuned to how symptoms of PMS affect your feelings, behaviour and your life. You may even find that self-monitoring your symptoms is an effective treatment in itself because it puts you in touch with your body instead of feeling let down by it. You may start to see your symptoms more realistically – only a few days of problems, for example – or you may home in on one particular problem – headaches, for instance – and be moved to find ways to treat it.

HOW TO FILL OUT YOUR DAILY CHART

Because we'd like you to fill out this chart for two to three months, we have provided three month-long charts at the end of this book. Each one has space for 31 days. (See Appendix 2.) It doesn't matter what day you begin charting, what matters is that you begin charting right now and continue to do so as you work through the 12-week plan. Don't think of recording as a chore. It is an important diagnostic tool to help you identify exactly when and how you are experiencing PMS and what can be done to alleviate your symptoms.

How the Chart Works

DATE
If you are menstruating, put a P after the date.
If you think you may be ovulating, put Ov after the date.

MEDICATION
Write down any medication you take that day. If you are on the Pill write that down too.

SYMPTOMS

List your symptoms. Mention both physical ones, for example headaches, and emotional ones, for example feeling depressed. Remember, you do not have to have a certain number of symptoms to have PMS. You may have more physical ones or just emotional ones.

DIET

You don't need to go into great detail here, but try to record your intake of fat, sugar, salt, caffeine and alcohol. Note down any food cravings you have in your comments for the day.

EXERCISE

Write down how active you were. It isn't just about going to the gym – even a 20-minute walk to the bus stop is worth putting down.

COMMENTS

Write any comments about your behaviour today. The evening is usually the best time to reflect on this. Just a few short sentences will do. If it was a good day, write that down. If you didn't feel productive or were easily upset or on edge, write that down too.

DAILY RATING

On a scale of 1-20, rate your overall mood for that day. Let 0 represent feeling on top of the world, and 20 represent a really bad day. A rating of 10 would indicate an average day.

EXAMPLE
Month # 1
DAY 1
Date: Nov 4
Medication: 2 Nurofen for headache
Symptoms: Bloating, breast soreness, headache, tearful, irritable
What did I eat today?
Breakfast: Toast, cereal, coffee

Lunch: Skipped
Dinner: Fish and chips. Ice cream
Snacks: 2 chocolate bars, crisps
Drinks: 2 glasses of red wine, diet coke, 3 cappuccino
Did I exercise today? No
Comments for today: Hungry for sweets. Tried to exercise but couldn't motivate myself. Felt fat and unattractive.
Daily rating: 17

DAY 2
Date: Nov 5 P
Medication: None
Symptoms: Fatigue and constipation
What did I eat today?
Breakfast: Cereal
Lunch: Tuna sandwich
Dinner: Baked potato, sausage and beans
Snacks: None
Drinks: 2 Cappuccino, 2 diet coke
Did I exercise today? Walked to shops, carried shopping home
Comments for today: Thank goodness my period came. Feel tired but happy
Overall daily rating: 3

I never used to keep a record of my menstrual cycle, which meant that I never had any idea when my symptoms might appear and when my period was due. A number of times I really thought I might be pregnant because all my symptoms suggested pregnancy. My breasts were heavy and sore. I felt a little sick and tired and I had to go to the bathroom all the time. I'd feel sensitive and lose my temper easily – but I didn't see this as unusual until my period arrived and then I could look back and understand what was going on. I could see that I shouldn't have panicked – I wasn't pregnant, I just had PMS. Now that I keep a record of my periods and when my symptoms are likely to occur I'm less likely to get into a panic. **Helen, 30**

In the sample below, can you see a general pattern of ups and downs and how they correspond with menstruation? The numbers stay lower than 10 in the early part of your cycle and get close to 20 as menstruation approaches.

Your PMS chart will help you identify those days when you are most likely to feel like comfort eating, giving up or snapping at someone. When you start to see a pattern it might be a good idea to mark those days in your filofax, dairy or planner to remind yourself that they may well come up and you need to stress-proof your life to cope with these symptoms.

If you are in a relationship it might help you and your partner feel more comfortable if your PMS chart was posted on the wall or fridge door. Mark for them the days when you are most likely to feel ticked off, not in the mood for socializing and so on so your partner can see what may be coming when. You could also encourage your partner to note down the differences they see in you on a monthly basis. You may be surprised to see it from their perspective.

> *If I told my girlfriend I thought she might be premenstrual she would fly off the handle. But when her GP suggested she fill out a chart she began to see that I wasn't insulting her or sweeping aside her feelings; she had a genuine problem that we needed to learn to cope with together.*
> **Martin, 26**

At the back of the book (after the three sets of blank 31-day charts in Appendix 2), you'll find your own PMS wall chart. It's repeated three times – one to use right now, one for 'his and hers', and one if you ever want to repeat the 12-week plan later as a booster plan.

Are You Sure It's PMS?

PMS is a sneaky set of symptoms that can be hard to pin down. That's why charting your symptoms, starting today, is so important. If you don't pay attention to the special characteristics and timing of your symptoms,

	Month 1 November	Month 2 December	Month 3 January
1	17		
2	18		
3	19		
4	16	20	
5	17	9	
6	18	18	
7	18	P12	
8	P15	P10	
9	P13	P9	
10	P12	P5	
11	P10	0	
12	P5	1	
13	0		
14	0		
15	0		
16	0		
17	0		
18	2		
19	0		
20	0		
21	Ov 3		
22	Ov 0		
23	14		
24	16		
25	7		
26	6		
27	1		
28	11		
29	16		
30	16		
31			

you may confuse them with other health concerns. You may, at this point, want to refer to Appendix 1, which lists a number of conditions that can often resemble PMS.

Lots of other conditions may have PMS-like symptoms, but there is an important difference: PMS only occurs in the run-up to your period, whereas non-PMS related conditions occur at other times in the month.

Getting Ready

If you feel your symptoms could be linked to other health problems, get them checked out and eliminated. Once you're sure it's PMS and have begun to chart your symptoms every day, the next step is to help yourself relieve the pain and discomfort you are experiencing. The 12-week plan is designed to help you do just that. But before you start the plan, give yourself a little time to get ready. The next chapter is all about preparing yourself so that you feel positive, energized and ready to start the 12-week plan and really give it your best shot.

Countdown: A week to get your mind focused for the best results

If you want to see positive results, you need to work with us for 12 weeks. That's quite a commitment, and the aim of this chapter is to help you get your head into gear so that you are less likely to give up and more likely to complete the plan. We recommend that you take a week to prepare yourself, ideally starting on a Monday. You can start on any day of the week you like, but it's assumed as you work through the plan over the next 12 weeks that Days 1 are Mondays and Days 6 and 7 are the weekends, with time for longer, more in-depth tasks. If you feel that you don't need as long as a week to prepare yourself, that's fine. Just make sure that you take enough time to focus on and prepare yourself mentally and emotionally for the weeks ahead.

A Week to Go

DAY 1

Starting today and for the next two to three months, make a commitment to fill out your symptom diary and PMS wall chart.

Keeping a health journal can be beneficial in many ways. Seeing things in writing can sometimes be an eye-opening experience! It may provide you with the motivation to improve your habits or cut down on those daily chocolate bars. It may also help you to identify what may be the cause of your problems or conditions. For example, you may notice that headaches always seem to occur after a pasta supper, or that more than four glasses of wine a day leaves you feeling exhausted the next. Your record-keeping may also prove to be useful to your doctor or health-care provider.

I began by keeping a chart of my symptoms, diet and exercise every day. This was quite revealing. After four weeks it actually became a straightforward system for monitoring my diet. I used a bright yellow highlighter pen to mark all those things I needed to avoid. The more yellow I saw, the more determined I got to improve my eating habits. The symptom chart taught me to really think about how healthy my lifestyle was. I didn't realize how many cups of coffee I was drinking and how little exercise I was actually getting. **Leah, 34**

This evening, after you have filled out your daily chart and given yourself a daily rating see if you can see any connection between your diet and exercise that day and the way you are feeling.

DAY 2

Talk to the people who are important to you about PMS. Ask them to support you and help you work through the 12-week plan. You are far more likely to be successful if you enlist the support of your partner, if you have one, and your family, colleagues and friends. Explaining to the people you care about why you are making lifestyle changes could not only help you; it could also encourage them to make positive lifestyle changes.

My partner is a great cook. Trouble is, he used to prepare dishes that didn't help my PMS. I had to tell him, which was tough, but he didn't seem to mind. He said he didn't like it when I was tired and moody, and if he could help he would. Now the food he prepares is much healthier and it tastes delicious. I feel better and I know he does, too. We both have more energy and are even thinking about joining a gym together. **Kim, 28**

Don't bottle up your feelings and try to cope on your own. Tell the important people in your life that you are starting a 12-week plan and ask for their support, encouragement and understanding. Make sure there are people you can turn to on the tough days, and people who will pat you on the back when you have good days. Your support network could make all the difference between living with PMS and beating it.

PMS is so common that you are bound to know someone who suffers too. You may want to think about working through the 12-week plan with together. That way you can keep each other motivated with regular discussion, updates and feedback. If you find it hard to talk about your symptoms with friends or loved ones, check out PMS support groups and websites (see the Maintenance chapter, page 263).

DAY 3

Do you have any time for yourself? This is probably more of a problem for women than for men. Women are more likely to be trying to do everything and be there for everybody: running a home, raising kids, being in a relationship and probably working as well. It's small wonder you have very little time for yourself.

Now is the time to clear your diary as much as possible to allow time to focus on you. This probably won't be easy, as you can't simply walk away from your commitments for 12 weeks, but there are ways that you can bring the focus back to you

Treat yourself to something today that you want. Buy a book or a magazine, get a new make-up bag or a new pair of shoes, or make sure you get to watch that TV programme you like. It doesn't have to be expensive, what matters is that you get used to spending some time and perhaps some money as well on yourself.

And get into the habit of booking regular time for yourself, when you do something just for you. Put it into your diary and treat it with the same importance as if it were a doctor's appointment. This is something you can't miss. Get your diary out right now and book yourself a treat for Day

6 or 7 this week. It doesn't matter what that treat is, just plan ahead for it. It might be a long bath, a massage, a manicure, a hair cut, a walk in the park or it could be a night away with your partner, going to the cinema or renting your favourite video. Think about what you would love to do but never seem to have the time for. It will give you a real lift to actually do it!

Over the next 12 weeks you will need to make sure that you have the space and the time on a day-to-day basis to read, think, write in your diary and go food shopping when you aren't hungry and likely to buy junk food. You'll also need time to eat and enjoy your food.

You also need to set aside a practical amount of time for daily exercise, starting with 10 minutes every day. Make that time when it suits you best. This may be when you get up, during the day or in the evening. You may need to be flexible. Whenever you do it, make time for it. It should be one of the most important things in your life over the next three to four months and, hopefully, once you realize how good it makes you feel this will encourage you to devote time to it for the rest of your life.

DAY 4

Think about what you hope to achieve from the 12-week plan today. It isn't enough to just want to get rid of PMS. That's only what you *don't* want. Figure out what you *do* want, how you want to feel, and work towards achieving that.

Personal trainer Pete Cohen, who has written several books on the subject of positive change, recommends doing this exercise to help you establish what your health goals are:

> Get a pen and paper and write down the first healthy goal that comes into your mind. You might write something like: 'I don't want PMS to take over my life' or 'I want to stop feeling bloated and heavy.' These are things you *don't* want. If you think about them your mind will dwell on these negative images. So try again.

> This time write down something positive. Something like, 'I want to look and feel great all the time' or 'I want to eat healthily all month long' or 'I want to be able to concentrate and feel in control of my life at all times.'

To beat PMS you need to think about how you will look and feel at the end of the 12-week plan. You could imagine how you would feel in three months time if you didn't do anything about it. Imagine how you would feel when you have yet another row over nothing with a friend or colleague at work. Imagine how you would feel if you put on yet another few pounds through comfort eating. Imagine how you would feel if yet another sleepless night cost you an important work contract or you overslept and were late to get your kids off to school. Imagine yourself. Would you look and feel good? Now imagine looking at your life in six months' time without any changes. Now in one year's time and two years' time. Do you like what you see? How many arguments have you had? How much junk food have you eaten? How much weight have you put on? How many opportunities have you missed out on?

Now try looking at it another way. Think about how you would look if you completed the 12-week plan successfully and were free of PMS. Really focus on how good you feel. How great it is to look in the mirror and like what you see. How great it is to feel in control. How great it is to feel energetic, healthy, sexy and vital all month long. Picture the new confident, healthy you in lots of situations: in front of the mirror, talking to your partner, family or friends, at work or just having fun.

Psychologists believe that to fix a new image in your mind, you need to repeat it at least 20 times a day. You are who you *think* you are and what you think about what you do. If you want to beat PMS for good, begin to fix an image of yourself living free from PMS in your head, starting today.

DAY 5

Are you the kind of woman who expects the best or the worst? Do you treat yourself with respect or are you hard on yourself? Do you think you will complete the 12-week plan or do you think you won't be able to beat PMS?

Make sure today that whenever you give yourself a hard time, you stop. Stop thinking that you are going to fail. Stop thinking that good things can't happen to you. Instead, start learning to expect to achieve your goals.

Your goals do need to be realistic. It's unlikely that you will look like you did when you were 16 again, no matter how hard you work. Nor, however much you imagine it, will you appear on the cover of Vogue. But you can look and feel your best. Make your expectations real and then stop thinking that you will fail. The 12-week plan is realistic, achievable and easy to follow. There is no reason why you should not succeed.

Start believing today that through the changes you make in the 12-week plan you will beat PMS, get your energy back and feel great all month long. Then expect to have achieved so much in those 12 weeks that you want to keep going with your new habits for the rest of your life. Expect to succeed. Use your imagination to reinforce this belief with the following visualization:

Find a comfortable place, close your eyes and relax. Be aware of your breath. As you breath in, think 'in', and as you breathe out, think 'out'. In, out, in, out. Each time your mind wanders off, follow it, observe that it has wandered, and then come back to your breathing. When you feel comfortable and relaxed enough, start to see yourself as healthy and happy. You look so successful and confident. Feel what it is like to be free of PMS. Make the vision as real as you can: see and hear the whole thing in glorious Technicolor, create the sound effects, feel the reality of your success. When you are ready concentrate on your breathing again, let your thoughts return, open your eyes and come back into the room.

If you have negative thoughts while you are visualizing, just let them go. Instead, see yourself succeeding. You use your imagination all the time. Why not use it to create success, good self-esteem and good health? Why not use it to beat PMS?

DAYS 6 and 7

On either of these two days, make absolutely sure that you relax and pamper yourself with the treat you arranged earlier in the week. Remember if you lead a busy life and don't organize time for you, then sooner or later your busy-ness will overwhelm you. Your life will be out of balance.

If you don't feel your best today, check to see if you are in balance:

- Have you had enough exercise today?
- Have you been in touch with your feelings today?
- Have you had enough mental activity today?
- Have you had time to think and reflect today?

You need to discover any source of imbalance and see what can be done to correct it. The 12-week plan can help you here. In addition to beating PMS, you'll find lots of suggestions and advice that can help you re-create balance, self-esteem and good health in all areas of your life.

Time to Begin

Hopefully, you will have found this preparation time useful. You feel relaxed, prepared and ready to beat PMS. All you need to do now is take a deep breath, turn the page and begin your journey towards a PMS-free life.

PART TWO

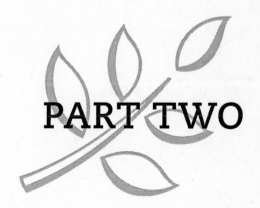

The 12-Week Plan

Week 1

At a Glance

DAY 1
Nutrition: Take the nutrient-deficiency quiz; throw out any foods in your cupboard that are going to make your PMS worse; do your PMS daily record and wall chart
Exercise: Assess your activity levels; go for a 10-minute walk
Emotional well-being: Start your emotional diary

DAY 2
Nutrition: Buy a multivitamin and -mineral supplement and start taking one every day; do your PMS daily record and wall chart; start to include phytoestrogens (soya) in your diet
Exercise: Go for a 10-minute walk and increase your activity levels in daily life; find out about local fitness classes in your area
Emotional well-being: Continue with your emotional diary

DAY 3
Nutrition: Your PMS daily record/wall chart; get used to reading food labels

Exercise: Go for a 10-minute walk and do some gentle stretching.
Emotional well-being: Think about the amount of 'me' time in your life

DAY 4
Nutrition: Do your PMS daily record/wall chart; re-read the information on good nutrition on pages 14–24
Exercise: Do your walk and your stretching; book yourself on a weekly fitness class
Emotional well-being: Make sure you have at least 20 minutes of 'me' time today

DAY 5
Nutrition: Do your PMS daily record/wall chart; read about the importance of magnesium in a PMS-busting diet
Exercise: Do your walk and your stretching and increase your activity levels in the day
Emotional well-being: Think of creative ways to spend your 'me' time

DAY 6
Nutrition: PMS daily record/wall chart; write out a shopping list and go shopping for healthy PMS-beating foods
Exercise: Go for a 15-minute walk and do your stretching
Emotional well-being: Plan a night out with your partner, a friend or someone you care about

DAY 7
Nutrition: PMS daily record/wall chart; try some home-made soup
Exercise: Be more flexible in your definition of exercise
Emotional well-being: Re-read your emotional diary and try a visualization exercise
VITALITY BOOSTER: Getting enough sleep

Day 1

NUTRITION
For each day of the plan over the next few weeks we will be giving you a
sample menu and a couple of tasks to think about. Whenever you see an
asterisk (*) after an item in the sample menu, you'll find the recipe in
Appendix 3.

You can stick to our menus if you want, or use them as guidelines to plan
your own menus. (If you are a Vegetarian or Vegan see 'Suggestions for
Vegetarians' below.)

The important thing is that you think about your food choices and how
they may be affecting your PMS.

Sample Menu
Breakfast: Slice of stoneground wholemeal toast with a scraping of butter
and boiled free-range egg, glass of fresh-pressed apple juice
Snack: Piece of fruit and small handful of fruit-and-nut mix
Lunch: Chicken with green bean and sweetcorn salad* or bowl of carrot
soup* plus pita stuffed with chicken or hummus and salad. Red fruit
based dessert – crumble tart or fresh fruit salad*
Snack: Vegetable sticks
Dinner: Roasted vegetables (tomatoes, mushrooms, aubergines (eggplant),
courgettes (zucchini) and new potatoes sprinkled with olive oil and
roasted at 180°C/350°F/Gas Mark 4 for 20 minutes), glass of red wine, dried
fruit (figs, apricots, prunes, apple) topped with low-fat yogurt

Suggestions for Vegetarians

It is important to make sure you get enough protein if you are a vegetarian. You need to replace animal protein with other food sources such as dairy products, pulses, legumes, nuts, seeds, grains and cereal otherwise deficiencies in vitamin B12 (almost only found in animal products, including meat and fish) vitamin D, calcium and iron are likely to trigger nutritional and hormonal imbalance and make your PMS worse. Here are some suggestions:

If you are the only vegetarian in your household make sure you substitute pulses, beans, wholegrain cereals, dairy products, tofu products or quorn instead of just leaving the meat part out of meals.

Choose cereals fortified with vitamins, especially B12. Try to eat a large portion of dark-green leafy vegetables every day and around a pint of whole or skimmed milk. If you are lactose intolerant you can get your calcium in calcium-enriched soy yogurts and milks or nut milks.

Eat dried fruits, pulses, green vegetables and wholegrains for fibre and iron. Cocoa powder and dark chocolate is a good source of iron, too.

Eat at least 30 g of pulses, nuts and seeds every day for protein and essential fatty acids. (EFAs)

Eat at least one serving of low-fat cheese or cottage cheese a day for protein and calcium – or a soya pattie or tofu portion.
Eat a total of three to four eggs a week.

Choose margarine or butter fortified with vitamins D and E in a vegetarian spread. You can get vitamin D from sunlight as well, and vitamin E from nuts and seeds.

If you are vegan you may need expert advice from a doctor or nutritionist. The Vegan Society websites have lots of useful info. Make sure you get enough protein and vitamin B12. The American Diabetic Association states that soy protein has been shown to be nutritionally equivalent in protein value to animal protein. Nuts, seeds, grains, pulses and vegetables are other good sources of protein. Yeast extracts used as food flavorings are often high in B12, but they are not high enough, and all vegans are advised to take a specific B12 supplement.

Task for Today

Take this nutrient deficiency quiz and read about the foods that contain the vitamins and minerals you might need.

Is your skin pale and unhealthy looking? Do you get bouts of acne?	You could be lacking in vitamin B6, vitamin C, Vitamin D and Vitamin E. You may also need more zinc in your diet.
Do you suffer from any of the following: mood swings and/or depression, sugar cravings, sleep problems, fatigue, poor concentration and low energy?	You could be deficient in the B vitamins, especially vitamin B6, and vitamin C and vitamin D. You may also need more calcium, magnesium, boron, chromium and iron.
Do you get breast tenderness?	You could be deficient in vitamin E, vitamin C, vitamin B6 and essential fatty acids (EFAs).
Do you get headaches?	You could need more vitamin B complex, especially vitamin B6, and magnesium and boron.

Do you get mouth ulcers, aches and pains? Do you find it hard to resist infection?	You could be deficient in vitamin C and calcium. You may also be lacking in iodine and zinc.
Do you suffer from water retention?	You could be deficient in B vitamins. You may also need more potassium, calcium and magnesium, or less sodium.
Irregular periods or problems with fertility?	This could be due to a lack of selenium and iodine.
Do you get muscles cramps? Are your teeth and bones healthy?	You may need more calcium and magnesium in your diet.

For what different vitamins and nutrients do for you, and the food sources of essential vitamins and minerals, see pages 267–71.

This week, buy – and start taking on a daily basis – a good multivitamin and mineral supplement. A good supplement can protect against the nutrient-depleting effects of stress and environmental toxins, and lack of certain vitamins and minerals may cause PMS or make it worse.

Since many experts believe that calcium and magnesium are the most important minerals for PMS, it is advisable to take them in a balanced formula separately from a multi-, as no multi- will contain adequate amounts of these two nutrients. 'In my experience', says nutritionist and PMS expert Ann Walker, 'most PMS symptoms will disappear by taking a Ca + Mg supplement alone – I recommend 1 or 2 Osteoguard or Osteocare per day, depending on whether the woman is taking any dairy produce or not.'

We talk more about the vital role calcium and magnesium play in your PMS beating diet plan later in the plan. However, be cautious when taking your supplements that you don't mix too many and end up taking more than you need.

Your final task today is to go through your cupboards and throw out all foods past their sell-by date, all processed and refined foods and hydrogenated fats. Look out for products such as ready meals, crisps, snacks and biscuits, but also margarines and low-fat foods, which often have lots of sugar added to make up for the lack of fat. We've listed below the kinds of foods you should be getting rid of, and the reasons why.

CUT THE CAFFEINE

'I can't start work without at least three cups of coffee,' says Ann, 38. 'I often have trouble sleeping, especially before my period and I need the pick-me-up.'

Caffeine is a stimulant that increases sleeplessness, anxiety and tension, which are all parts of the PMS problem. It can be found in coffee, tea, soft drinks and chocolate and some over-the-counter pain-relievers. Even decaffeinated drinks contain some caffeine.

A study[1] of over 200 college-age women found severe PMS symptoms in 60 per cent of those who drank more than four cups of caffeinated drinks a day. We know that even tiny amounts will stimulate the release of adrenaline, which isn't good news if you have PMS. And coffee is metabolized slowly – even one cup of coffee or a soft drink at dinner may stop you sleeping well. Coffee also causes your body to get rid of important nutrients, especially B vitamins that are needed to fight PMS.

It's best to cut out caffeine altogether, especially if you get PMS breast tenderness, but if you can't do that, at least cut down in the two weeks before your period. Just cutting back on your intake can make a positive difference. Aim for two or three caffeinated drinks a day, maximum. Taper it off gradually, and withdrawal symptoms such as headaches should not last more than two weeks.

SHUN THE SUGAR

I had extreme sugar cravings and it wasn't unusual on a bad day to get through a whole packet of chocolate biscuits and then eat another packet an hour later. About an hour after eating the treats I'd feel really depressed and eat more chocolate. It was a vicious circle. **Sharon, 20**

I knew a bit about diet but I had no idea that cutting down on my sugar intake would bring me back to normal and get rid of my PMS, and that's what it has done. I now know that sweet things make me feel depressed and of course I put on weight and get PMS too. Knowing this makes them much less appealing. **Cheryl, 37**

Like caffeine, sugar perks you up, then drops you with a bang – not what you want if you're already feeling low with PMS or fighting fatigue. Remove as much sugar as you can from your diet, because research shows that the more you eat, the less likely you are to get your full quota of vitamins and minerals.[2] Sugar has many different names, including dextrose, fructose, lactose, maltose and sucrose. If you see more than one of these names on your food packets, the food may contain more sugar than you thought. If sugar is the first ingredient listed on a cereal box, get rid of it and replace it with one that has wheat or oats as the first ingredient.

AVOID ALCOHOL

When my PMS is really bad I think 'What the hell, a little wine will take the edge off my symptoms.' Unfortunately, I soon find myself drinking more than a little, and drinking even when I don't have PMS. **Carol, 30**

Drinking alcohol will make your symptoms worse, especially in the two weeks before your period when your body is more sensitive to its effects. It interferes with hormonal function and the proper absorption of B vitamins and magnesium. Alcohol can also cause low blood sugar by blocking the body's ability to supply glucose when it is needed. And to top it all, alcohol is a depressant.

The best strategy for the next 12 weeks is to avoid alcohol altogether, but if you do want to drink, do so as an occasional treat, drink only with a meal and try to drink when you aren't feeling premenstrual. The rest of the time, try non-alcoholic drinks like sparkling mineral water with a slice of lemon, fresh-pressed juice diluted with spring water or alcohol-free beer or wine.

Once you have eliminated PMS, you can drink alcohol in moderation again. Try not to drink every night, but if you do, two glasses of wine is your absolute maximum.

CUT DOWN ON SALT

Salt (sodium chloride) holds water in the body tissues and contributes to PMS bloating and water retention. Even if you don't have problems with water retention, it's still good to limit your salt intake, as excess sodium can cause high blood pressure which later in life can cause strokes and other health problems.

Almost everything you eat – except natural unprepared foods like fruits and vegetables – has salt added. The hidden salt adds up quickly. In place of salt you can use lemon juice or vinegar on vegetables and salads, and fragrant fresh herbs like basil, rosemary and coriander in your sources and salads. Try spices and dried peppers on your popcorn.

FAT

Limit your intake of saturated or hydrogenated fats, and make sure you get enough essential fatty acids (EFAs). If you eat too much saturated fat it occupies the cells and spaces in your body where EFAs should go – not good for PMS acne, breast tenderness and bloating. Lots of high-fat foods, such as hot dogs, hard cheeses, crisps and cakes, are also high in salt and sugar, which won't make you feel good. Cutting down on saturated fat will help ease PMS symptoms, and you'll have more energy and find it easier to manage your weight.

EXERCISE

Take time out of your day for exercise – walking, biking, jogging or whatever you enjoy. For the next 12 weeks, think of exercise as a preventative medicine. You are relieving pressure and tension – both psychological and physical – before they build up.

According to Professor Steven Blair at the Cooper Institute in Dallas, being unfit – rather than obesity – is linked to poor health and PMS. Unfit slim people have a death rate double those who exercise regularly.

Walking vigorously is a form of aerobic exercise. Aerobic exercise helps to stabilize blood sugar and raises your level of feel-good hormones. It also reduces stress. If you are the kind of woman who is always in high gear and your mind is constantly racing, walking can help calm you down. Walking also gives you time for yourself. For best aerobic results, use your arms and go as fast as you can without losing your breath or breaking into a jog.

Look at your day and see if you can fit in 10 minutes or so, and then treat your walk as seriously as you do your other duties and appointments. Apart from responsibilities to those you care about, what can be more important than doing something to get rid of premenstrual symptoms?

EMOTIONAL WELL-BEING

Dr James Pennebaker, a Professor in the Psychology Department of Southern Methodist University in the US, has documented the powerful healing effect of writing down your feelings. It not only boosts your mood, it improves your physical health.

So find a small notebook you can easily carry around, and spend a few minutes each day recording your emotions. Ask yourself:

How did I feel when I woke up?
How did the day ahead seem?
How did I feel after breakfast?
How did I feel in the morning?

How did I feel after lunch?
How did I feel in the afternoon?
How did I feel after supper?
How did I feel about my day before going to bed?

If you find it difficult to express your feelings, try to spend a little time each day writing about the most stressful events in your life today – or the most traumatic circumstances of your past. Write a diary, a poem, a story or whatever becomes your way to feel free and safe to illuminate what is inside. You may want to express your emotions in picture form. There is no right or perfect way to express yourself. That is the beauty and magic of it. What works for you may not work for someone else. The important thing is that you find a way to express your emotions and feelings every day.

Day 2

NUTRITION

Sample Menu
Breakfast: Take your supplement with a breakfast of wholegrain cereal, skimmed organic milk or calcium-enriched soya milk with chopped and or dried fruits on top, plus a glass of fresh-pressed apple juice.
Snack: Small flapjack
Lunch: Tuna salad with soy nuts,* wholegrain roll, rice dessert*
Snack: Piece of fresh fruit and small handful of fruit-and-nut mix
Dinner: Stir-fried vegetables (a good colourful mix – peppers, onions, garlic, ginger, bean sprouts, carrots, celery, mushrooms) with grilled chicken breast or marinated tofu pieces; banana surprise*

Task for Today
Include phytoestrogens in your diet. One of the most potent phtyoestrogens, called genistein, is found in soya products. Soya is especially good for PMS, and you'll start to notice it in our sample menus.

Phytoestrogens come in two forms: isoflavones and lignans. You can get isoflavones in soybeans and soy products such as soymilk, soy flour, tofu, miso and natto. Lignans are found in whole grains, linseed (flaxseed) and, in lesser amounts, in apples, celery and parsley.

You can also find phytoestrogens in certain plants: black cohosh, licorice root and fennel.

The best way to increase the amount of phytoestrogens is to eat a diet rich in plant foods – vegetables, fruit and whole grains. Try also to eat a couple of servings of soy-based food a week. Soya beans are easy to cook and delicious when added to salads, soups or bakes. Soya yogurts or milk added to carbohydrates have a refreshing and pleasant taste. Tofu in thin slices can be added to stir fries, or whizzed in a blended smoothie. Tempeh is great grilled in a sandwich. Start getting used to buying and eating soya-based products. Not only do they taste great, they are good for you, too.

EXERCISE

Make a real effort today to be more active than you usually are. Be more active around the office, if you work outside the house, or at home. Don't overdo it, just gently increase your activity levels.

Moderate Activities You Could Build into Your Life
- walking a couple of bus stops
- parking further from work/shops
- walking or biking instead of sitting in traffic jams
- using the stairs
- washing the car yourself
- doing some gardening or DIY
- spring-cleaning your house
- taking a dog for a walk
- cleaning the windows
- cancelling deliveries and walking to the shops for milk and papers

Do your brisk 10- or 15-minute walk. Choose a different route so you don't get bored.

Spend some time today finding out about classes in your local area that you might like to join, for example dance, swimming, yoga, tai chi. If you don't want to join a class, think about joining a gym or swimming pool or buying a home exercise video.

EMOTIONAL WELL-BEING

Fill in your emotional diary again today, and before you go to bed re-read what you wrote yesterday. Note any similarities and differences from yesterday in the way that you feel. Start to think about your emotions as feelings that pass over you, not as feelings that identify who you are. Just because you feel sad does not mean you are a sad person. The important thing is not that you felt an emotion, but how you responded to it. Did you let sadness or anger control you, or did you find ways to manage it and direct it positively?

Day 3

Sample Menu
Breakfast and multivitamin: Fruit salad including a small banana, sprinkled with chopped nuts, glass of calcium-enriched soya milk, or nut milk or organic semi-skimmed milk
Snack: Handful of mixed seeds and a piece of fruit
Lunch: Greek salad* yogurt treat*
Snack: Small pack of twiglets and piece of fruit
Dinner: Grilled chicken or fish or tofu/bean burger and big green salad (cucumber, mixed leaves, spring onions, peppers, shredded crunchy cabbage) with new potatoes, garlic, lemon juice and hemp/pumpkin seed oil dressing, apple crunch*

Task for Today
Today's task is to read and understand labels on the foods you have left in your cupboards to see if there are any surprises that should have been chucked out. It's not always just the obvious culprits that contain fats, sugar and salt, etc. Food labels often don't make it clear, and all these ingredients can go by other names. Here's a checklist of what you should be looking out for:

- Sodium is salt
- Animal fat is saturated fat
- Transfatty acid is another name for hydrogenated fat
- Sugar has lots of pseudonyms: sucrose, fructose, dextrose, corn syrup, malt syrup, maple syrup
- Artificial sweeteners to be avoided include: mannitol, sorbitol, xylitol, acesulframe K, saccharin and aspartame.
- Colourings: artificial colour added, FD and C red no 3, the words green, blue or yellow followed by a number, tartrazine (E102), quinoline yellow (E104), sunset yellow (E110), beetroot red (E162), caramel (E150)
- Safe additives that you don't need to throw out include: annatto, green chlorella and carotene.
- Preservatives: Citric and absorbic acid are natural substances which are OK, but synthetic additives like BHA and BHT are not. Alum or aluminum, sodium nitrate or other nitrates, monosodium glutamate (MSG) and sodium inosinate, sulphur dioxide and sulphites, and benzoic acid and benzoates should also be avoided.
- Emulsifiers, stabilizers and thickeners: Some of these are quite harmless, for instance lactic acid, guar gum, calcium chloride and fumaric acid, but a good rule of thumb when choosing food is to avoid products whose chemical ingredients outnumber the familiar names. If you can't understand a label and there is barely enough room on it for all the chemical ingredients, avoid it.

EXERCISE

Go for your 10- or 15-minute walk, try to be more active in general and start doing some stretches. Stretching improves your flexibility and is a good way to relieve stress, ease muscle pain and increase relaxation, all of which are important in the battle against PMS.

Stretching should be done slowly and carefully to avoid injuring the muscles. When you assume a stretching position, stretch as far as you can without straining too much and hold it for 30 to 45 seconds. Towards the end of the time, try to stretch just a little bit more, hold for a few moments and relax.

Stretching can be very relaxing, but do take care. Take the time to learn the correct way to stretch from a professional, for if you stretch incorrectly or bounce instead of gently holding a stretch, you could do more harm than good.

Some Simple Stretches

CALF STRETCH
Lean against a wall or press your heels down on a step.

THIGHS
Stand by a wall or chair with your knees together, then bend one leg at the knee and hold it by the heel behind you.

HAMSTRINGS
Lie on your back with both knees bent and the soles of your feet on the floor. Keeping your back on the floor and the other knee bent, grasp your leg with your hands around your thigh and gently stretch it towards you.

LOWER BACK
Lie on your back and draw your knees into your chest.

WHOLE BACK
Kneel on all fours with your knees under your hips, your arms under your shoulders and your back straight. Round your spine, tucking your tailbone underneath you and relaxing your head and neck to stretch your back. Return to neutral, slightly arching your spine with your head up.

NECK AND SHOULDERS
Try some shoulder shrugs and neck roles and circles.

WAIST
Try a gentle side stretch with both knees bent.

ARMS
Try holding your arms in front of you and imagine you are holding a big beach ball.

STOMACH

Lie flat on your front and rise on your elbows, bringing your shoulders back and pushing your hips down to feel the stretch in your stomach.

WHOLE BODY

Put your hands in the air, rise up onto your toes and stretch upwards as if you were trying to reach the stars.

EMOTIONAL WELL-BEING

If you don't take the trouble to look after yourself and recharge your batteries, who will?

There are two different ways to recharge your batteries. You need one or two hours a week of complete relaxation, and you also need shorter 10- to 20-minute breaks every day or every other day. Either way, they should be 'me' time – time that you spend on yourself.

If you were given an extra two hours a week on the condition that you would use it only for yourself, how would you use it? Write down the top three things you would like to do, and then look at your wish list. Do the things you have listed have anything in common? For example, are they related to study, outside activity, pampering, peace or a hobby?

Decide whether you would benefit from a planned hour on a regular basis doing the same thing – for example, an evening class. Or you might prefer a different activity each week – perhaps a walk one week, the cinema the next or reading. Now imagine that you have to book that 'me' time each week in your diary. How about marking that hour or two in your diary right now for the next 11 weeks?

Now that you have booked in your hourly slot, try to build daily 10- to 20-minute slots into your day of relaxation. This isn't a waste of time – you will be so much more efficient when you start your regular activities again than if you had worked through this period.

During your 10- to 20-minute break try to do things you want to do – for example, phone a friend, read the newspaper, listen to your favourite song, take a shower or bath. For these few moments, try to avoid pleasing anyone but yourself. Don't feel guilty about doing this. You are not doing anyone any favours if you overdo it and become irritable. Just a few minutes for you every day can make all the difference between coping and losing it.

Day 4

NUTRITION

Sample Menu
Breakfast with multivitamin: Scrambled egg on wholegrain toast plus a glass of fresh-pressed apple juice
Snack: Glass of calcium-enriched soya, nut or semi-skimmed organic milk and a piece of fresh fruit
Lunch: Bowl of lentil soup* and tuna or egg or hummus and salad sandwich
Snack: Sesame snaps or oat rice cakes plus four dried apricots or dates
Dinner: Chicken, tofu or bean burger with big mixed salad and small baked potato; baked apples* stuffed with raisins and served with low-fat vanilla yogurt

Task for Today
Re-read the information on Good Nutrition (pages 14–24) at the start of the plan to refresh your memory on how the food choices you make can help or hinder PMS.

EXERCISE

Continue being a little more active than usual. Go for your 10-minute walk and do some stretching to relax you.

Ring up and find out how often the classes you fancy run and how much they cost, and book yourself on one for next week or the week after.

EMOTIONAL WELL-BEING

Keep filling in your diary and thinking about the way you feel. Don't forget to give yourself that mini-break at some point today. Note in your diary how you feel before and after your 'me' time.

Day 5

NUTRITION

Sample Menu
Breakfast and multivitamin: Wheatbran cereal topped with low-fat yogurt and sprinkling of chopped nuts with soy milk, nut milk or semi-skimmed milk, glass of fresh-pressed apple juice
Snack: Dried apricots and crackers
Lunch: Tofu with pasta salad* slice of pumpkin and raisin bread*
Snack: Handful of mixed seeds and a piece of fruit
Dinner: Dark green leafy vegetables, new potatoes, beans and peas with fish; stewed fruit with low-fat vanilla, strawberry or chocolate yogurt

Task for Today
Today we are going to turn the spotlight on magnesium and its crucial role in easing PMS symptoms.

Magnesium is vital for almost every bodily process. It is needed to convert fat, carbohydrate and protein into energy and to regulate blood sugar. It works alongside calcium to perform many of its functions, so a deficiency in magnesium can affect calcium metabolism, too.

As far as PMS is concerned, magnesium helps to reduce water retention, improves glucose tolerance and eases menstrual headaches and migraines.

Many women with PMS have very low levels of magnesium.[3] Luckily magnesium supplements can help.[4] In one study, women with PMS were give 360 mg of magnesium three times a day. Their symptoms improved within two months. Another study showed a significant reduction in water retention in women who took 200 mg of magnesium every day for two months.

Your body needs a steady supply of magnesium. Foods rich in magnesium include wheat bran, wheat germ, whole-wheat flour, nuts, beans, peas, dark green leafy vegetables, dried fruit, fish and tofu. In our Sample Menu for today we have deliberately included lots of magnesium-rich foods. It might also be a good idea to start taking a supplement, as your multivitamin and -mineral won't contain enough and magnesium is essential if you have PMS.

So how much magnesium should you have? The recommended daily dose for women in the UK is 270 mg. Many PMS experts recommend large doses – say 400-800 mg for women with PMS. Too much magnesium may cause diarrhoea, so you should begin by taking 200 mg and then increase to 400 or more if your body copes well.

Magnesium's healing powers are magnified by vitamin B6, calcium and potassium, so make sure your multivitamin and -mineral supplement contains those too. In general supplements do not contain a lot of potassium. You need to get this from fruit and vegetables. Taking magnesium in the form of magnesium oxide is not so well absorbed as magnesium in the form of citrate or asparate.

EXERCISE
Do your walk and stretching routine and continue to think of ways to increase your general level of activity throughout the day.

EMOTIONAL WELL-BEING
Be creative today with your 'me' time. Learn to see opportunities in places you wouldn't normally – take a book to read on the bus, daydream in the bank queue, listen to your favourite music when you cook your tea, use a special body lotion after your shower or spray on that favourite perfume for the day.

Day 6

NUTRITION

Sample Menu
Breakfast with multivitamin and -mineral and magnesium: Skimmed or soya milk porridge with chopped bananas and nuts plus glass of fresh-pressed apple juice
Snack: Piece of fruit and small raisin biscuit
Lunch: Avocado and salad sandwich on wholegrain bread plus small slice of chocolate cake*
Snack: Glass of milk plus fresh fruit
Dinner: Wholemeal pasta with vegetables (onions, broccoli, sweetcorn, tomatoes) and topping of grated cheese, fresh fruit and nut salad*

Task for Today
Today is the day to stock up on healthy foods. Prepare a list of food you have enjoyed from this week. Plan your menus for the week ahead, and make a list of the ingredients you will need. Try to leave out anything with sugar, caffeine, artificial sweeteners, preservatives or additives and convenience foods in general.

You might want to think about buying the following essential store cupboard ingredients:

- Fresh fruit and vegetables, organic dairy produce, including live yogurt, free-range eggs and unhydrogenated margarine, lean meat, oily fish and soya (not to be put in your store cupboard, as they need to be eaten within a few days, but an essential for your weekly shop)
- Wholemeal rice, oats, millet
- Whole wheat pasta
- Wholemeal flour
- Whole meal crackers, bread, rye bread
- Cans of beans and pulses with no salt or sugar added – lentils, chickpeas, kidney beans
- Sea salt or rock salt with no chemicals added

- Honey, maple syrup, barley malt or apple juice for sweetening
- Nuts and seeds
- Dried fruit in moderation. For example raisins, apricots, dates
- Cold-pressed vegetable oils, such as sesame and sunflower oils (try extra –virgin olive oil for cooking)
- Low-salt stock cubes
- Herbs, spices and vinegar for flavouring
- Breakfast cereal and porridge – don't forget to read the label
- Coffee substitutes – such as grain coffee
- Tea substitutes such as herb teas, fruit teas, green tea
- Unsweetened pure fruit juice, diluted. Avoid flavored mineral water, squash and fruit drinks
- Soy milk, yogurt and tofu products such as sausages

EXERCISE

Again, do your walk and your stretches. If you have been walking briskly for 10 minutes, increase that to 15. Clear your diary for the next 11 weeks with your chosen night of the week to exercise based on the class you want to try, or the exercise video or bike or treadmill you'll use at home and so on, and tell everyone that this is your exercising night.

EMOTIONAL WELL-BEING

Arrange for you and your partner or a friend to go for a walk or a meal, a coffee or a drink to relax and chat about how your week is going with the plan.

Day 7

NUTRITION

Sample Menu
Breakfast and multivitamin and -mineral and magnesium: Wholemeal muffin with teaspoon peanut butter and sliced banana, glass of milk and herbal tea
Snack: Baked potato filled with hummus or tuna and sweetcorn plus bowl

of salad and seasoned steamed vegetables, yogurt dessert*
Snack: Wholegrain rice cakes or oatcakes with organic low-fat cream cheese and handful of grapes
Dinner: Chicken and vegetable curry with steamed basmati rice (excuse for a takeaway); fruit-based dessert

Tasks for Today
Reread the nutrient-deficiency quiz on pages 54–5. Familiarize yourself again with which foods boost magnesium.

Your last task this week is to treat yourself to some home-made soup. Soup is a staple part of any diet and it is also rich in goodness and fibre, and low in salt and additives. Home-made soups retain the maximum goodness of their ingredients, which makes them the best health bargain for women with PMS. Not only do you get a bowl full of vitamins and minerals, sugar-balancing protein and energy-giving carbohydrates, you benefit from phytonutrients.

In Appendix 3 you'll find some soup recipes, but we are sure you can come up with some of your own. Tomato and lentil, potato and carrot, leek and onion, noodle soup – the possibilities are endless. Freeze what is left over in case you don't have time for a full meal in the week.

EXERCISE
Read the chart below to see that exercise doesn't have to be about sweating it out in a gym. Being an active partner in sex, doing vigorous housework, dancing and other everyday activities can all help boost health.

Activity Calories Burned per Hour

Running 6 minutes a mile	1,000
Running 9 minutes a mile	750
Swimming, fast	600
Squash	630
High-intensity aerobics	520
Swimming, moderate	460

Rowing machine	440
Dancing, fast	440
Tennis	400
Low-intensity aerobics	400
Walking, fast	390
Cycling, 10 miles an hour	380
Badminton	370
Gardening	300
Hiking	370
Cycling, 5 miles an hour	250
Dancing, social	170
Cleaning windows	120
Vacuum-cleaning	135
Dish washing	60
Making love (depending on how vigorous)	100 - 400

EMOTIONAL WELL-BEING

Read back through your diary and look at the range of emotions you can go through in just seven days. Look through your diary and try to work out when things from outside your control affected you and when things came from inside you. Do you notice any patterns?

There are techniques you can use to change your reaction to things over which you have no control. Whenever you notice yourself getting stressed – for example if you are stuck in a traffic jam, or the next queue in the supermarket moves more quickly than yours, or the cashpoint isn't working – try to think about how important it really is in the scheme of things. Put it into perspective. You could also try this visualization when life gets too busy and you feel everyone is making demands on you:

When you have a few minutes to spare, find a quiet, private place and sit down and relax. Close your eyes and become aware of your breathing. When your mind and body are feeling deeply relaxed, create in your imagination a beautiful scene. Choose an outdoor setting by the beach, in the mountains, in a garden – wherever you like. Fill the scene in with colour and detail and create your own wonderful holiday snaps. Let the details of the place sink in, see the sights, smell the fragrances, hear the birds singing, the running water, and the waves crashing. When you have created your own little paradise, slowly return to the room and open your eyes.

Now you can go on holiday anytime you like. There's no packing, no queuing and it's free!

VITALITY BOOSTER

Getting Enough Sleep

If you are not getting enough sleep you could find yourself depressed, irritable, tired and grumpy. Sounds like PMS, doesn't it? You are in fact less likely to get a good night's sleep before your period, because during the PMS phase your serotonin/melatonin (hormones that promote a good night's sleep) levels drop. Because of this you could end up in a vicious circle – PMS causes sleep problems, and too little sleep makes PMS worse. So what does lack of sleep do to us? One important study[5] looked at the effects of inadequate sleep (four hours or less a night) on the blood sugar levels of women with PMS. The study found that after a week of restricted sleep, the body's ability to secrete and respond to insulin, which helps regulate blood sugar, had dropped significantly. The researchers reported that the decrease in insulin response was almost identical to that reported among people with diabetes.

Research has also shown that the ageing process is increased in people who are sleep-deprived. Poor sleeping habits also lower the immune system, meaning that you are more likely to get colds and flu, increases stress and irritability, contributes to memory loss and concentration problems and, of course, makes you feel tired.

So it is important you get good-quality sleep of between 6 to 9 hours every single night. How can you do that?

STEP ONE: BOOST YOUR SEROTONIN

The first thing to think about is boosting your serotonin levels. If your serotonin levels are high, you will feel happy and calm in the day, and when night comes serotonin will convert to melatonin and you'll sleep soundly. When you wake up, melatonin will convert back to serotonin and you'll feel like leaping out of bed. If you've got PMS the chances are that you are low in serotonin/melatonin.

Fortunately you can eat foods that boost your serotonin (and by extension your melatonin) supply. Serotonin is manufactured within your body from the amino acid tryptophan, and is found in many foods – notably eggs, cheese, milk, lean meat, fish, soybeans and potatoes. That's why the old advice to drink a glass of warm milk before you sleep can work wonders. You can, if you prefer, take tryptophan in supplement form from healthfood shops. You might also want to consider adding a couple of crackers or a slice of bread to your bedtime snack to help you sleep well. This is because complex carbohydrates such as rice, oats and wheat encourage insulin to be released, and when insulin is released tryptophan is, too.

In order for tryptophan to convert to serotonin it needs vitamin B6, so you need to ensure that you have enough vitamin B6 in your diet. You can get B6 from foods such as spinach, fish, lentils, avocados, carrots and potatoes. Increase your vitamin B6 supplements in the premenstrual period, especially if you find you feel depressed at this time.

You also need to get plenty of exposure to light. Light is necessary for serotonin production. Get some light each day, or consider buying a light box.

Finally, any food that is rich in minerals – especially calcium, magnesium and silicon – induces a calming action in the mind, and a deficiency can lead to sleep problems. Try to include more of them in your diet. Foods rich in these minerals include watercress, broccoli, parsley, leeks, spinach, almonds, sesame seeds, sunflower seeds, dried figs, pulses, beans, lentils brown rice, peaches, bananas, dates, avocados, raisin and sea vegetables.

STEP TWO: GOOD SLEEPING HABITS

Most of the time I sleep like a log but when I have PMS I have real trouble getting to sleep or if I do fall asleep I find myself wide awake at 2 a.m. I hate feeling so exhausted the next day. **Lisa, 35**

Whether you struggle with falling asleep or wake in the middle of the night (most typical for women with PMS), some basic good sleep strategies will help you to regain control. These include:

- Stick to a regular sleep-wake pattern, even on weekends. Ideally you should aim to be in bed around 11 p.m., as studies show that people who sleep before midnight tend to wake more refreshed than those who go to bed in the small hours.
- Decide how much sleep you need. Eight hours is enough for most people, but you may need more or less to feel alert and refresh. If you want to nap during the day, research shows that 25 minutes is the optimum time for a nap.
- Make sure your mattress and bed are comfortable. Use your bed for sleeping and sex only, so that you only associate it with rest and pleasure when you get into bed. Block out noise and light, as light will impair the production of melatonin. Sleep in a well-ventilated, cool – but not cold – room (around 55-65°F/12-17°C), as body temperature naturally falls at night.
- Wind down for an hour or so *before* you go to bed. Activity delays melatonin production. Try taking a nice bath, doing yoga, having a quiet chat, making love, doing relaxation exercises, or drinking a cup of camomile tea. If you can't sleep after lying in bed for more than half an hour, get up and do something monotonous like reading or ironing. Then when you feel sleepy, go back to bed.
- It isn't wise to eat a heavy meal or drink a lot before night-time. Stay away from caffeine and alcohol. Besides disrupting your sleep, alcohol can trigger PMS symptoms.

OTHER HELPFUL TECHNIQUES

You might want to add aromatherapy oils, such as lavender or bergamot, to your bath. Dead Sea salts, which contain potassium and magnesium, can have a therapeutic effect on body and mind. Or sprinkle a few drops of lavender essential oil on your pillow, or have a gentle massage with the oils.

Herbs can help with sleep problems. Valerian, hops, passionflower, camomile and skullcap all work as gentle sedative and can improve the quality and duration of sleep. White chestnut Bach Flower Remedy calms the mind and instils an air of tranquillity.

Many women take magnesium tablets to help them sleep better. Magnesium is often called nature's own tranquillizer and, as we have seen in this week's nutrition plan, it helps relieve PMS symptoms, too.

Visualization techniques can help if you find it hard to switch off from the day's events. Focus your mind on something that is relaxing, your dream location or happy memories, and you may find it easier to let go of the day.

Try acupressure. There is an acupressure point on your body called Heart 7 whose main action is to calm the mind and alleviate insomnia. Trace your little finger down the inside of your wrist to the crease where Heart 7 is located. Gently rub the point using your thumb for around 1 minute. Breathe deeply while you do this and feel peace and tranquillity flowing into your body and mind.

Practise some relaxation techniques. Try lying on your back in bed, tensing every part of your body in turn and then relaxing it. This way you can feel how good it is to relax. You might want to do this accompanied by some relaxing music.

Avoid long daytime naps, which can cause fragmented sleep or insomnia. An hour before you go to bed, write a 'to do' list for tomorrow and put out the clothes you want to wear to stop you mulling over what you need to do and wear tomorrow.

If none of the above works, try not to get upset. Keep things in perspective. The more you worry about not sleeping, the less likely you are to sleep well. And the chances are that if you sleep badly one night, you'll sleep like a log the next, especially if you are doing your daily exercise.

Week 2

At a Glance

DAY 1
Nutrition: Eat healthily and take your multivitamin and -mineral and magnesium; your PMS daily record and wall chart; focusing on the importance of calcium in your PMS busting diet
Exercise: Do your 15-minute walk and increase your activity levels
Emotional well-being: Take an honest look at the amount of stress in your life

DAY 2
Nutrition: Eat healthily and take your multivitamin and -mineral and magnesium and calcium; do your PMS daily record and wall chart; think about the amount of caffeine in your diet
Exercise: Plan a fun activity with a loved one this weekend that involves exercise; do your 15-minute walk and stretching routine
Emotional well-being: Identify your stress triggers

DAY 3

Nutrition: Eat healthily and take your multivitamin and -mineral and magnesium and calcium; do your PMS daily record and wall chart; avoid caffeine until noon
Exercise: Do your 15-minute walk and stretching routine
Emotional well-being: Think about new ways to cope with stressful situations

DAY 4

Nutrition: Eat healthily and take your multivitamin and -mineral and magnesium and calcium; do your PMS daily record and wall chart; avoid caffeine from noon until 5 p.m.
Exercise: Do your 15-minute walk and stretching routine and have a little dance
Emotional well-being: Try some of our stress-busting tips

DAY 5

Nutrition: Eat healthily and take your multivitamin and -mineral and magnesium and calcium; do your PMS daily record and wall chart; avoid caffeine after 4 p.m.
Exercise: Do your 15-minute walk and stretching routine
Emotional well-being: Try some breathing exercises

DAY 6

Nutrition: Eat healthily and take your multivitamin and -mineral and magnesium and calcium; do your PMS daily record and wall chart; try to go for one full day without caffeine; think about buying a juicer and try some alternative drinks
Exercise: Get active with a friend or loved one this weekend and have fun exercising or walking together
Emotional well-being: Discover the delights of massage

DAY 7

Nutrition: Eat healthily and take your multivitamin and -mineral and magnesium and calcium; do your PMS daily record and wall

> chart; cooking methods that include more raw food in your diet
> *Exercise*: Try exercising for 20 minutes
> *Emotional well-being*: Try some of our stress-management
> techniques
> *VITALITY BOOSTER*: Boosting your energy levels

Day 1

NUTRITION

Sample Menu

Breakfast and multivitamin and -mineral and magnesium: Fruit salad sprinkled with chopped nuts, slice of wholegrain toast with scraping of butter, glass of calcium-enriched soya milk or organic skimmed milk

Snack: Small flapjack

Lunch: Lean meat or fish or low-fat cheese, medium jacket potato, cheese, cucumber, red pepper and orange salad*

Snack: Vegetable sticks

Dinner: Vegetable soup* slice of wholegrain bread with scraping of butter, berries topped with low-fat yogurt, glass of diluted fresh-pressed apple juice

Task for Today

Today the spotlight is on calcium and why, along with magnesium, it is crucial if you have PMS.

A 1998 study at St Luke's Roosevelt Hospital in New York[1] on 466 women with moderate to severe PMS symptoms showed that after three months those taking a 1,200-mg calcium supplement experienced significant improvement in their symptoms in comparison to those who got the placebo.

Additional research[2] shows that women with PMS have disturbances in the way their body regulates calcium during the second half of their menstrual cycle. Why does this happen? No one knows for sure.

Undoubtedly the anti-inflammatory effects of calcium and its role in the production of serotonin play a part. Whatever the reason, when calcium levels in the body fall too low in the premenstrual period, PMS is more likely to occur.

Make sure from now on as you work through the plan that your diet is rich in calcium, especially in the two weeks before your period. Non-fat dairy products such as calcium-enriched skimmed or semi-skimmed milk, and low-fat cottage cheese, are good sources of calcium. Spinach, tofu, collard greens, almonds, fish with bones such as salmon or sardines, oats, sesame seeds, soybeans, broccoli, nuts, pulses, root vegetables and leafy green vegetables are all sources of calcium.

If you have PMS there may be no alternative but to supplement, especially if you don't eat much dairy. The recommended daily intake for a woman in her reproductive years is around 700 mg. The best type of calcium supplement to take is calcium citrate because it is easily absorbed, but it is also OK to take calcium carbonate as long as some dairy products are taken to aid absorption (lactose aids absorption).

It is always advisable to take magnesium if supplementing with calcium, as the two minerals complement each other. The jury is still out on the exact proportion of calcium to magnesium that is most beneficial. For most people it appears that 2 parts calcium to 1 part magnesium is fine, but those with particular problems with magnesium status may require a ratio of 1:1. It would be advisable for someone with PMS who does not take much dairy produce to supplement 800 mg of calcium and 400 mg of magnesium. Halve this if your dairy intake is reasonable but not up to target intakes. Make sure that your diet and your multi-vitamin and -mineral includes sufficient levels of vitamin D, as without vitamin D your body can't absorb the calcium you ingest.

Finally, foods that are high in fats and/or sugars will inhibit calcium absorption. Avoid alcohol, caffeine, junk food, excess salt, sugar and white flour. If you stick to our healthy eating guidelines you shouldn't have a problem eating foods that will help calcium do its job well.

EXERCISE

If you have signed up for an evening class, sport or activity or bought a home exercise video, this week is when you will probably start. If your class is today, you don't need to do your allotted walk or stretching for the day. If it isn't today, increase your walk to 15 minutes and do your stretching. If it's raining or cold outside, wrap up warm – or find somewhere where you won't be disturbed, play some upbeat music and dance for 15 minutes. The important thing is that you just move your body.

If you are in a relationship, why not initiate sex this week? 'When you have PMS,' says Lucy, 40, 'sex is off the menu more often than it is on. I'm pleased to say that it's me chasing him these days. We enjoy regular sex now, just as we did in the days before PMS. It's great for both of us.'

EMOTIONAL WELL-BEING

Today we would like you to focus on how damaging negative stress can be. It can trigger PMS symptoms, stop you coping and make your symptoms worse by interfering with hormonal health.

When you are stressed, adrenaline is released from the adrenal glands. Adrenaline, as you know, has a blocking effect on progesterone and can result in premenstrual symptoms. If you have been under continual stress or your blood sugar levels have been fluctuating, your adrenal glands may become exhausted and won't be able to produce normal amounts of cortisol and other hormones. Give your adrenal glands a break and find ways to manage stress effectively.

You are already working on eating well and exercising more. And last week we focused on getting enough sleep. The next thing is to try to keep the effects of stress from interfering with your hormonal health. Tomorrow we'll be doing some work on identifying your stress-triggers.

Day 2

NUTRITION

Sample Menu
Breakfast with multivitamin and -mineral and magnesium and calcium: Oat-based cereal with calcium-enriched skimmed milk, glass of fresh-pressed apple juice
Snack: Sesame seed biscuits
Lunch: Broccoli soup*, Salmon fish cake*, organic new potatoes, serving of spinach with scraping of butter
Snack: Handful of nuts and raisins
Dinner: Vegetable risotto*, hot fruit with low-fat calcium-enriched yogurt

Task for Today
Today we would like you to turn your attention to the amount of caffeine in your diet.

The best thing to do is to try and cut caffeine out of your diet completely, but if you can't live without your latte or your diet cola, at least cut back your consumption in the week or two before your period, since it takes longer for your body to break down caffeine in the premenstrual days.

Start to avoid caffeine today. If you are used to drinking more than two cups of coffee a day or a couple of caffeine-containing beverages a day, it isn't a good idea to cut them out straight away. Caffeine narrows your blood vessels and if you suddenly stop your blood vessels will widen and you will get splitting headaches. Take it easy and cut back gradually. This week drink no more than 2 cups of tea or coffee a day and start substituting a glass of water at the other times, supplemented with a slice of lemon to give it a sharper taste. Or try decaffeinated teas, coffees and soft drinks, or grain-based coffee such as Postum or Caffix, or refreshing herbal teas. Or substitute diluted fresh-pressed juices or smoothies.

EXERCISE

Do your 15-minute walk and stretching routine and invite your partner or a friend or family member to something that is active and fun this weekend. It could be a disco, ice skating, a funfair, a city walking guided tour, a walk in the country, a ballroom dance class, a house party, or a game of netball or football. Exercise doesn't have to be about gyms and 'no pain, no gain'. Exercise can be a lot of fun. It is a wonderful way to lift your mood. Research[3] shows that exercise releases brain chemicals called endorphins, which can help you feel happier, more alert and calmer. These endorphins can have a dramatic and positive effect on PMS depression, anxiety and mood swings. Exercise[4] can reduce stress, raise self-esteem and improve mood. It can be even more rewarding if you enjoy it with friends or loved ones. That way you can support each other, spend more time together and have someone to discuss your progress with.

EMOTIONAL WELL-BEING

What makes you feel anxious and tense? Identify your stress triggers and write them down. What makes you stressed? Here are a few thoughts to get you going. Tick some in the list below and then add some more of your own if you like:

- [ ] your partner
- [ ] your family
- [ ] your job
- [ ] your house
- [ ] commuting
- [ ] your kids
- [ ] your friends
- [ ] your appearance
- [ ] your finances
- [ ] your responsibilities at home, or work or to others
- [ ] little things like junk mail, ansaphones and cash points with no cash
- [ ] politicians
- [ ] your boss

☐ your colleagues
　Other things that really tick me off:
☐ ....
☐ ....
☐ ....
☐ ....

You may find that only a few things get you stressed, or you may have a long list of stressors. Whatever it says on your list, just make sure that you start homing in on what is causing problems in your life. Until you know what is stressing you out, it's hard to find positive solutions.

Now think about the impact stress is having on your health. What symptoms of stress do you display? Don't forget that if they appear all month long they are not PMS but stress-related.

☐ Tendency to get colds and flu and infections
☐ Headaches
☐ Irritable bowel
☐ Irregular periods
☐ Mouth ulcers
☐ Mood swings
☐ High blood pressure
☐ Pain in shoulders and back

Now that you have a clear idea of what your stress triggers are and the way you respond to them, you can start thinking about dealing with them. If you don't know why you are stressed or you don't think there is anything you can do, talk to your GP or someone you trust. You may also find that counselling or psychotherapy can help you to explore ways to cope better with stress. One idea is to take the test on the website for the International Stress Management Association: www.isma.org.uk. Tomorrow we'll take a look at taking the first step in stress-beating.

Day 3

NUTRITION

Sample Menu
Breakfast with multivitamin and -mineral, magnesium and calcium: Wholegrain
cereal with fresh fruit, seeds and skimmed organic milk, glass of fresh-
pressed apple juice
Snack: Handful of dried fruits, seeds, nuts
Lunch: Lentil chilli*, fresh fruit and almonds
Snack: Wholemeal scone with low-fat cottage cheese
Dinner: Steamed fish or tofu with organic brown basmati rice and stir-fried
vegetables in ginger and garlic; bowl of berries with low-fat or soy yogurt
and crushed amaretti biscuits on top

Task for Today
Try going until midday without any caffeine, and try two drinks you
haven't tried before as alternatives – from herbal or fruit teas to
decaffeinated coffee.

EXERCISE
Do your 15-minute walk then find some stairs and complete 1 minute of
walking up and down them. Use the second hand on your watch to time
you or, if you haven't got a second hand, count slowly to 60. Then choose
two stretches – perhaps the calf stretch and the hamstring stretch – and
hold each for 60 seconds. As you feel the stretch ease off, slowly increase
the stretch. Then walk up and down the stairs for another minute. Finish
with the full-body stretch and hold for 1 minute.

EMOTIONAL WELL-BEING
Often when we feel stressed it feels as if the situation is out of our hands,
but you don't have to let stress damage your physical and emotional
health. You can make changes in your life that put you back in the driver's
seat. You can get back in control.

Whatever is causing you stress, focus today on ways that you can change the situation for the better. You won't be able to make these changes overnight; the important thing is that you stop hoping the problem will go away and start thinking about what you can do and what positive changes you can make. Then, over the weeks ahead, start to make these changes – by downsizing, moving, working at home, getting extra help with the house or children, reorganizing your finances and priorities and putting your energy more into your health and well-being than in material things. The stress isn't going to get any better unless you do something about it. This may not be easy ,but it is important that you persevere. If you can keep your stress load to a manageable level and do something to limit it when it threatens to get out of control, not only will you feel better, your symptoms will improve, too. Tomorrow we'll explore some stress-busting tips.

Day 4

NUTRITION

Sample Menu
Breakfast with multivitamin and -mineral and magnesium and calcium: Poached free-range egg on wholegrain toast, piece of fresh fruit, glass of calcium-enriched soya milk
Snack: Packet of twiglets, some dried apricots
Lunch: Potato and vegetable salad* or Spanish omelet*, fruit tartlet
Snack: Low-fat yogurt with chopped banana, sesame seeds and nuts
Dinner: Vegetable soup* with a veggie sausage or lean chicken/seafood sandwich with green leafy vegetables, fruit and oatcakes dessert

Task for Today
Drink no more than 1 or 2 cups of caffeinated products in the morning, and then try going all afternoon without any caffeine. Once again, try drinks you haven't tried before as alternatives.

EXERCISE

Do your 15-minute walk and some stretching. Sort through your CD collection. Make sure you have enough dance music to keep you going if the weather gets too cold, windy or rainy to do your walk.

EMOTIONAL WELL-BEING

Sometimes, though, however hard we try, we can't change a situation that is stressful. The phone keeps ringing, the kids keep arguing, the traffic is impossible. Your heart starts to beat faster and you feel tense. What matters now is how well you cope with the stress. What coping strategies do you use? Do you let it overwhelm you or do you find ways to deal with it?

If you feel that your coping strategies aren't as effective as they could be here are some practical stress-busting tips you might want to use in stressful situations:

1. *Breathe In*
This belly-breathing exercise will help you beat stress.

> Stand up or lie down and place your hands, one on top of the other, 3 cm (about 1½ inches) below your navel. Breathe out, imagining the air flowing into the area beneath your hands. Visualize a positive energy flowing from this area, up your arms and back round into your tummy with each breath. Repeat this breathing until you feel relaxed.

2. *Release the Tension*
Do you hunch your shoulders when you are stressed? Do you tighten your fists? Do you cross your arms? Do you wrap your legs around each other? Become aware of the way your body reacts when you are under stress. Then, whenever you feel yourself going into that stress position, do the opposite – release your shoulders, stretch out your hands, uncross your arms or legs, and don't forget to breathe.

3. Unwind in the Bath

Why not try a bath with essential oils? Jennie Harding, essential oil therapeutics tutor from the Tisserand Institute in the UK, believes that baths with essential oils are aromatherapy's answer to stress. When you feel tense, try one of the following:

- 3 drops patchouli and 3 drops sandalwood
- 3 drops rosewood and 3 drops clary sage
- 2 drops vetiver and 2 drops jasmine

If your skin tends to get dry, put the oils into half a teacupful of full-cream milk, then add this to the water.

4. Get the Hankies Out

Whenever you feel tense, 2 or 3 drops of lavender oil, relaxing ylang ylang or calming camomile dropped on a hankie and then inhaled can help calm you down. Or you might like to try 2 drops of peppermint or lemon essential oil on a tissue and inhale when stressed. If you prefer you could also burn these oils in a vaporizer to help clarify and invigorate your mind.

5. Herbal Relief

One of the best herbs for relieving tension is camomile, as it has a gentle sedative effect. Drink a cup of camomile tea anytime you feel tense. If you drink a cup before you go to bed, this can help you sleep. Hops are also good as they relax the nervous system. Pour a cup of boiling water onto a teaspoon of dried hops and leave to infuse for 15 minutes before drinking.

6. Flower Power

Bach Flower Remedies can help you relax. Put a few drops on your tongue in an emergency, or diluted in water as directed. Try olive for relaxation, aspen for panic or Rescue Remedy when your brain is screaming for it all to stop.

7. Massage
Have a shoulder or Indian head massage to help you relax – it's blissful - more about the delights of massage on pages 94–5.

8. Stroke Your Pet
If you have a pet, stroke it. It's been proven to lower blood pressure and stress levels. If you haven't got a pet, why not give someone you love a hug? It will have the same effect (just don't tell them they're your new pet!).

9. Stop Frowning
Relax your jaw by gently resting the tip of your tongue for a second behind your top front teeth. At the same time, try to consciously relax your facial muscles and let your shoulders drop down and away from your ears by an inch or two – you'll be amazed to realize how you were holding that tension in your body.

10. Stretch
Whenever you feel stressed, the full-body stretch (page 65) can help you unwind. Yoga postures are excellent for stretching out tense muscles and promoting breathing and relaxation. Try these poses:

COW HEAD STRETCH
Sit on the floor with your heels tucked under your bottom and breathe regularly. Reach over and behind your right shoulder with your right hand, keeping your elbow pointing up and your arm close to your ear. With your left hand, reach behind your back from below and try to interlock your fingers (don't worry if you can't). Hold for 30 seconds, breathing deeply, then repeat, alternating arms.

KNEE PRESS
Lie on your back, legs outstretched with your arms at your sides. Exhale and bend one leg towards you, hugging the knee into your

chest. Hold the position for a few minutes, breathing normally.
Inhale and release the leg, lowering it slowly to the floor. Repeat
slowly with the other leg.

11. Write it down

When it all seems too much, grab a pen and paper and write down what
you need to do. Listing things on paper will help to focus your mind,
enabling you to think clearly about what is a priority, what can wait and
what can be delegated to someone else. Once a job has been dealt with, be
sure to cross it off the list. Watch your list shrink!

Day 5

NUTRITION

Sample Menu
Breakfast with multivitamin and -mineral and magnesium and calcium: Sugar-
free baked beans with wholegrain toast, piece of fresh fruit, glass of
diluted fresh-pressed apple juice
Snack: Low-fat digestive biscuit, tea or coffee with skimmed milk
Lunch: Pesto*; fruit-based dessert such as baked peaches, or a crumble
Snack: Vegetable sticks with low-fat cottage cheese
Dinner: Spicy vegetable stew*, 2 slices wholemeal bread with meat or fish
or tofu and salad; small bar of organic dark chocolate

Task for Today
Today, try to make sure you drink no more caffeine (i.e. tea, coffee, soft
drinks, chocolate) after 4 p.m. Once again, substitute drinks you haven't
tried before as alternatives.

Re-read the notes on calcium (page 269) to familiarize yourself with foods
that are rich in it.

EXERCISE

Do your 15-minute walk and your stretching routine.

EMOTIONAL WELL-BEING

Spend 5 minutes when you get up and 5 minutes before you go to sleep doing a basic breathing and relaxation exercise. The way you breathe actually affects the way you think, feel and act. Most of us breathe around 12 to 18 times a minute. If you can reduce your breaths to 8 a minute or fewer, this will automatically increase your feelings of self-esteem and control.

> **The Basic Breath**
> Sit on the edge of a chair, back straight and feet on the floor. Hold your hands around your lower abdomen, one each side of your stomach with the backs of your hands resting on your thighs. Exhale fully with a loud sigh. Deflate your stomach down to your groin and hold it empty for a few seconds. Start to inhale very slowly with your mouth closed and feel your lower abdomen swelling in your hands. Visualize the area from your groin to your rib cage as a beautiful coloured balloon and watch it inflate slowly, filling from the bottom. Expand your balloon fully and hold for 3 seconds. Exhale slowly, watching the balloon deflate until your abdomen is flat. Repeat this exercise 10 times.

Day 6

NUTRITION

Sample Menu
Breakfast and multivitamin and -mineral and magnesium and calcium: 1 slice of rye toast with caraway seeds, low-fat yogurt, glass of freshly squeezed orange juice
Snack: Dried fruit and sesame seed crackers with low-fat cottage cheese

Lunch: Spinach salad with tofu*, fresh fruit salad
Snack: Wholemeal scone with low-fat spread, glass of calcium-enriched soymilk
Dinner: Baked potato, broccoli and beans dinner*; baked apples stuffed with raisins and cinnamon

Task for Today

You may have already managed a morning, an afternoon and an evening without caffeine. Are you ready to go for a whole day with any caffeine at all? Don't worry if you don't feel ready yet. Keep cutting back on your intake and make sure that, at some point over the next 11 weeks, caffeine-free days start to become more routine.

Have you experimented with alternative drinks?

Remember that water is vital for your hormone systems to function at their best. If you don't drink enough water you start to feel tired, dizzy and could get headaches and stomach upsets. Aim for 6 to 8 glasses or 1½ litres/2¾ pints of fresh water a day. (This sounds a lot, but don't forget that fruits and vegetables count towards your fluid intake as they are around 90 per cent water.)

Fill a pitcher or a bottle with your targeted amount of water and drink it throughout the day. Take it with you in the car, to work – just keep it nearby. If the bottle is empty by bedtime, you have achieved your goal. Fresh juice is another excellent way to increase your fluid intake. Not only is it a great substitute for caffeine, but by extracting the juice from fruit and vegetables you provide your body with an excellent source of nutrition that is easy to digest and therefore can be assimilated by your body almost immediately.

There is also another benefit to raw juice: It has a laxative effect. So start gently! Watch out for juice drinks that are expensive fakes packed with additives and preservatives and that number-one PMS enemy: sugar. Try some of the better-quality juices, squashes and cordials and fruit teas. (They aren't really teas at all, but just use the name as they are infused with hot water.)

Alternatively, purchase a juicer and squeeze your own. Fresh and ripe fruit should be used, ideally at room temperature. Wash it using cold running water before you put it though the juicer. According to health and fitness guru Leslie Kenton, raw juice once exposed to the fresh air will start to deteriorate, so drink it immediately. Appendix 3 offers some juice recipes to get you going.

EXERCISE

Go dancing or do whatever you planned (on Day 2) what you would do at the weekend. Hopefully your partner or friend will keep you company and you can both have lots of fun. And don't forget it's your chance to be the active partner in sex this weekend.

EMOTIONAL WELL-BEING

Do your breathing exercises again. We'd also like you to consider the benefits of massage for stress-reduction.

Massage

Massage is perhaps one of the oldest and most influential therapies. It is very effective in dealing with stress, relaxing the central nervous system, improving the circulation and encouraging the body to get rid of toxins. For instance, a recent study at Toronto Hospital found that a 15-minute massage for the nurses significantly reduced tension and improved mood and relaxation. Other great benefits include: improved circulation, stimulation of a sluggish metabolism, decreased blood pressure, increased levels of endorphins, toxin-removal, improved sleep and pain relief.

Why not book yourself in for a massage at the weekend? Local sports centres or health clubs will usually have a resident masseur. You could ask for a whole-body massage or you could have a massage for areas of your body that suffer most from tension, such as your back and shoulders. Indian head massage has been used as a stress-buster for thousands of years, relieving tension in the thin layer of muscle surrounding the skull. For PMS the most helpful kind of massage is probably Swedish massage. The skin and muscles are gently stroked with extra pressure on tight, knotted areas.

To work on specific areas that are causing tension you may want to try Shiatsu, which involves pressure placed on various points of your body to break up and release energy blockages. Make sure the massage is comfortable – if it feels too rough or doesn't make you feel good, tell the masseur or masseuse, he or she will welcome the feedback.

DIY Massage Techniques

Place your hands gently on your face, palms over your eyes.

Hold the side of your head to help relieve tension. Use your whole hand to press gently with your palms just above your ears, your fingers meeting in the middle of your forehead. Then let go. It is actually the sensation of pressure and then letting go which is relaxing. Pressure should be light – the aim is to hold, not press.

Put both hands behind your neck and gently interlock your fingers. Then gently rub the sides of your neck with your palms to relieve tension in the neck and shoulders.

Day 7

NUTRITION

Sample Menu

Breakfast and multivitamin and -mineral and calcium and magnesium: 1 slice wholegrain toast with cottage cheese, 1/4 cup of blueberries and a handful of toasted almonds
Snack: Low-fat yogurt with chopped nuts
Lunch: Carrot, orange and tomato salad* with lean meat or fish; gooseberry fool
Snack: Dried fruit and packet of twiglets
Dinner: Cheese and vegetable bake*, dried fruit compote*

Task for Today

Today we would like you to think about the way you cook your food. Cooking limits the effectiveness of the nutrients we eat. For example, it is thought that around 50 per cent of B vitamins are lost through cooking, and we know how important they are if you have PMS. And some experts, like Dr Viktoras Kulvinskas, author of *The Survival Report into the 21st Century*, estimates that we may lose as much as 85 per cent of nutrient value when we cook.

Overcooking food doesn't help our bodily systems, either. Digestive problems can result when you eat and drink food that is too hot. A study published in the *Lancet* reported that 77 per cent of people who drink tea above 137°F/58°C had stomach upsets. In another study reported in the *Lancet*, overly hot food was linked to an increased risk of mouth ulcers and tongue and throat cancers.[5] Perhaps even more worrying is the conclusion drawn by Dr Edward Howell, who devoted a lifetime researching the effects of a diet full of cooked food. He linked a cooked food diet to a reduction in brain tissue and the swelling of key organs.

On top of all that, cooked foods may also weaken the immune system. A research paper was presented by Dr Paul Kouchakoff at the first International Congress of Microbiology called 'The influence of cooking food on the Blood formula of man'. The paper reported that eating cooked food weakens the immune system. The end result is that you get sick more, or simply feel tired and run down all the time.

This may all sound alarming, but don't panic – there is good news. At the same International Congress, Dr Kouchakoff also suggested that eating an approximate ratio of 50-50 raw foods to cooked foods, heated below 190°F/85°C, could prevent this risk to the immune system.

An all-raw food diet isn't advisable, since our systems can't handle that. But this week, increase the amount of raw or lightly cooked foods you eat. Aim to eat some every time you eat cooked foods. And when you do cook, cook gently at a lower heat, letting your food simmer or steam lightly. When cooking fruits and vegetables it is better to warm them rather than vigorously cook them. (A good trick when making soups is to heat the soup and then at the last minute add some raw vegetables which are just warmed by the soup broth.)

Here's an overview of cooking methods that preserve the nutritional status of the foods we eat, and other methods that may result in a substantial loss of essential nutrients.

Steaming	This is the best way to cook vegetables because a higher proportion of essential vitamins and minerals are preserved than when the same items are boiled. Vegetables also taste crisper and fresher after they have been steamed, unlike boiled vegetables which can go soggy and tasteless.
Stir-frying	A good and very quick and easy way to cook a wide variety of foods, including fish, lean meats and vegetables, without adding a large amount of fat.
Poaching	This is a clever way to lightly cook fish, and a good alternative way to cook eggs.
Grilling	Ideally grill on a rack that allows the fat to drain away in the cooking process.
Roasting	Always the best way to cook meat, since other methods such as frying use too much fat.
Deep-frying	Always to be avoided because this method of cooking uses a high proportion of fat.
Boiling	Not the best way to cook vegetables because too high a proportion of nutrients leach into the liquid during the cooking process. If you do boil vegetables, keep the water to add to soups and sauces. Please note, however, that there are some ingredients, such as dried beans and pulses, which have to be boiled in plenty of unsalted water until they are fully cooked.
Creamy sauces and salt	Avoid dishes that involve the addition of rich sauces, and avoid the temptation to add salt when cooking. You don't need it. Use herbs and spices instead.

Microwaving   We do not yet have any clear idea of the effects of eating
               microwaved food, and we do not know what molecular
               changes may be happening to the food when cooked. Best
               to limit as much as you can.

Why is raw food so good for us? The bottom line is it provides us with a
broader range of nutrients than any other way of eating. Raw fruits and
vegetables are packed with vitamins and minerals, have enough protein
and are low in fat. They are rich in slow-releasing carbohydrates that
boost energy, and fibre that improves digestion. But the truly remarkable
thing about raw foods are the enzymes they contain.

Enzymes are essential for all biochemical and physiological functions in
your body. We depend on them to walk, talk, breathe, eat, sleep and fight
illness. They are released as soon as we start to chew, and they are the
keys to proper food absorption and the quality of your health. As soon as
we cook or even freeze foods, we start to destroy the enzymes. That's why
it's important to gently cook your food – with the exception, of course, of
meat and fish, and raw beans and pulses, which should always be cooked
thoroughly.

Here are a few examples of postive benefits of raw foods:

Linseeds   Assist in hormone-production and the health of the
(Flax seeds)   reproductive glands
Celery   High in B vitamins that can promote relaxation and
               restful sleep
Roquette   Can boost energy production
(arugula)
Tomatoes   Assist digestion
Courgette   Helps cleanse bodily organs
(zucchini)
Parsley   A great immune-booster

Sprouts

If PMS leaves you feeling run-down, tired and moody, perhaps the most energizing and beneficial raw food choice is sprouts.

One of the greatest studies ever conducted in the field of natural health was supervised by Dr Edmond Bordeaux Szekely over a period of 33 years, during which time he evaluated over 120,00 people regarding the experimental effects of eating raw foods. He identified the most life-enhancing, high-energy, nutrient-rich foods as sprouts.

Sprouts refer to the seeds of legumes and grains that have been germinated for three to five days into small plants. Each sprouting seed has enough nutritional and life-force to grow into a full healthy adult plant, and that is why they have more nutritional activity than any other raw food – because they are, in effect, still in the process of growing.

Millet and quinoa seeds are often thought to have the most therapeutic effect for mind and body. In addition to these grains, wheat, rye, oats, barley, seeds, nuts and pulses can also be sprouted. You can easily sprout seeds and beans at home. All you need is a jam jar, your seeds or beans, fresh water and a piece of cheesecloth.

1 Rinse the seeds well. Place in a jar and cover with a few centimetres of boiled water.
2 Cover with a piece of cheesecloth secured with elastic band and leave overnight in a warm dark place.
3 Rinse the next day with fresh water and drain well and return to the dark. Do this until the seeds start to grow. Then place them on a sunny windowsill for a few hours.
4 Eat them now or store in an airtight container in the fridge. They will keep in the fridge for a few days.

You can also buy sprouting kits from your health food store or mail order (see Resources chapter).

If you aren't used to eating raw foods, or haven't sprouted at home before, it might take a while before you get into the habit. Give it time. Over the next 11 weeks, gradually increase the amount of raw food you eat – remember the ideal ratio is around 50 per cent raw to 50 per cent cooked.

Eating more raw food needn't be scary. Your salads, fresh-pressed juice, fruits and vegetable-stick snacks already count. Now stir some sprouts into you home-made soup, sprinkle bean-sprouts raw onto your stir fry instead of cooking them, and eat lots of fruit snacks. You get the picture. After a month or so you'll be amazed at how dramatically your energy levels, PMS symptoms and all-round health improve.

EXERCISE

Do your stretching and go for a 20-minute walk. There is something magical about the 20-minute mark. Twenty minutes of exercise – preferably every day, but at a minimum of three times a week – has:

    a positive effect on blood flow
    makes your heart and lungs grow stronger
    gives you more flexibility
    strengthens your bones
    improves your posture
    enhances your self-esteem
    enhances your sex life
    helps with weight-management
    reduces stress
    improves mood
    has a beneficial effect on PMS.

If you are finding it hard to motivate yourself, remind yourself of all the great things exercise can do. It really is good for you, we promise!

EMOTIONAL WELL-BEING

Don't forget to fill out your emotional diary for this week. Have a think once again about what your stress triggers are – you listed them on Day 2.

And repeat the following to yourself several times a day and whenever you feel tense:

I can cope with stress. I am calm and in control.

Write this down and put it up somewhere visible. Make it your mantra. Then try three of the tips for stressbusting from Day 5 – choose the ones that appeal to you the most. Make a note in your emotional diary how you feel before and after using them.

VITALITY BOOSTER

Boosting Your Energy Levels

It's hard to explain, but when I have PMS there are times when I feel as if the life has been sucked out of me. I know that even if I get my 8 hours I'm not going to feel that much better. My eyelids feel so heavy and tired, and everything, even thinking, is an effort. I don't just feel sleepy or tired – I could deal with that – I feel completely drained. **Sonia, 37**

If your energy levels have a habit of dipping below zero, this week you can find and cut out the things that are draining your mental, emotional and physical vitality. PMS may make you feel run-down, but as you'll see below, it isn't entirely to blame.

The 10 Most Common Energy-drainers and What You Can Do About Them

1. SUGAR
Is your diet too high in sugar or food with little or no nutritional value? When you feel tired, do you reach for a chocolate bar or something sweet and comforting? Sugar is also a nutrient-robber, washing away vital supplies of B vitamins and chromium. Deficiency in B vitamins and chromium can lead to fatigue and diabetes. Opt for snacks such as fruit and nuts, and sweeten food with dried fruit such as dates. Eat biscuits made from wholemeal flour to make sure you get B vitamins and chromium and to give you a more consistent burst of energy.

2. CAFFEINE

Caffeine can, like sugar, interfere with blood sugar; it is especially important to avoid caffienated drinks with a meal, as they contain substances that can inhibit the absorption of zinc and iron by up to 50 per cent. Iron-deficiency can lead to anaemia, and carbonated drinks like cola can leach calcium from your body. It's best to avoid caffeine, but if you must drink it wait at least an hour after eating a meal before you have a caffeine drink.

3. ALCOHOL

The odd glass won't harm you, but drinking too much disrupts the absorption of many vial nutrients, including B vitamins, magnesium, zinc and iron. A lack of any of these nutrients can cause fatigue. Alcohol also contains high levels of sugar and can contribute to mood swings, blood sugar problems, depression and insomnia.

If you do drink a little more alcohol than intended, up your intake of B vitamins from good food sources such as grains, dairy, nuts, fish and eggs. It might also help to keep a diary so you can see how much you are drinking. Try also to keep two or three days of the week totally alcohol-free. When you do have some alcohol, sip your drink slowly and stick to smaller measures. Don't get influenced by other drinkers. If you find it hard to cut down, confidential advice is available from some of the organizations listed in our Resources chapter.

4. SMOKING

Cigarette smoking depletes nutrients in your body, especially vitamin C and E, both of which can boost vitality. But smoking doesn't just drain your energy levels. It can also make PMS worse.

Studies have shown that smoking can have a negative effect on your hormones, it reduces oestrogen levels and has been linked with infertility and early menopause in women. Smoking also leads to high levels of cadmium, which can stop the utilization of zinc, a mineral that is crucial for the health of your reproductive system. When you are on the 12-week plan, it is a good idea to avoid anything that can upset the delicate balance of your hormones.

Let's cut to the chase here. The health risks of smoking are well known, and if you want to beat PMS and improve your health and well-being, you need to stop smoking. It's best to avoid nicotine gums or patches, as these can become addictive. It's also best if you feel strong enough to go cold turkey: set a day and a time to smoke your last cigarette and then become an ex-smoker. If you need help, try acupuncture or hypnotherapy. It's also a good idea to plan ahead for those times in the day when you feel most tempted to smoke. Contrary to what many believe, it is not nicotine smokers miss (nicotine clears out of your body within 48 hours) but the habit of smoking itself – so find other ways to end a meal, to relax, unwind or deal with your nerves.

If you are an ex-smoker or passive smoking is an issue, you may need to think about increasing your intake of vitamin C. The vitamin C needs of smokers are thought to be double those of non-smokers at 100 mg a day. Make sure you eat the recommended five portions of fruit and vegetables a day.

HELP FOR SMOKERS
QUIT is a UK charity dedicated to offering help to people who want to stop smoking (see the Resources chapter). Here are QUIT's tips for stopping smoking:

1 Make a date to stop smoking and stick to it.
2 Throw away all your cigarettes and ashtrays. Keep yourself busy to help you get through the first few days, and make sure you drink lots of water throughout the day and night.
3 Be more active. This will help you relax and take your mind off smoking.
4 Think positive. The discomfort and cravings are positive signs that your body is recovering. They usually only last a week or two.
5 Change your routine. If you always smoke after a meal, make sure you have a book or magazine on hand. If you always smoke at the pub, go somewhere else for a while.

6 Don't make excuses - a celebration or a crisis is not a good reason to have just one quickie.
7 Use the money you save to treat yourself to something nice.
8 Watch what you eat. Replace fatty foods with fruit if you feel hungry.
9 Take one day at a time and remember, every day without smoking is good news for your health.

For extra support, call a helpline (for example, QUIT on 0800 002200). This will put you in touch with someone to talk to on the phone or a local support group.

5. STRESS

As we have seen, the hormones released in stressful situations deplete the body of essential nutrients such as magnesium. Effects of magnesium deficiency include difficulty relaxing, insomnia, muscle spasm and fatigue. If life feels stressful, pay attention to the magnesium levels in your diet. Good food sources include oats, green leafy vegetables and sesame or sunflower seeds. A daily portion of each will help you get the RDA of 300 mg.

6. ANTIBIOTICS

Antibiotics destroy illness but they can also destroy friendly bacteria in your intestines, leaving yeast and fungi such as *Candida albicans* to thrive – which is why thrush often occurs after a course of antibiotics. Candida may also produce toxins that can reduce the absorption of nutrients, causing fatigue. If you get an infection, only take antibiotics if they are absolutely essential. A good wholefood diet with plenty of fruit and veg helps prevent infections in the long term, and if you do get an infection Echinacea supplements and vitamin C have antibiotic effects.

7. LACK OF SLEEP

Nothing makes you feel more drained than consistently poor sleep. Re-read the notes on sleep in Week 1. If you are under stress it is essential to get around 8 hours of good-quality sleep each night.

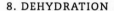

8. DEHYDRATION

Check your fluid levels. It's hard to drink enough water each day and much easier to stock up on dehydrating tea and coffee. Most people need about 2 litres of hydrating fluid a day. What you are aiming for is pale yellow urine.

9. WORRY

Negative thought-patterns sap energy. Changing your perspective from negative to positive can change your whole physical feeling – we'll explore this more in Week 3. If your mind is buzzing with worries, imagine your thoughts are like rain running down a window ledge. This will help clear your mind of the negativity that can sap your energy.

10. REPETITION

Doing the same thing for hours on end can sap energy. To boost your energy levels, try not to do any one thing for more than 90 minutes. This is the optimum amount of time that you can perform well at any task. Anything will do to change the pace – a cuppa, a chat with a friend or, best of all, a brisk walk and some fresh air. It's well known that lack of natural light and exercise are big energy-sappers.

If you feel tired all the time, you may need to check with your GP or a health practitioner to check for an underlying problem such as anaemia, underactive thyroid gland, glandular fever or depression.

Here are some additional boosters you might like to experiment with this week:

FUEL FOR THE BODY

The best foods for ensuring a sustained energy release are complex carbohydrates. Choose wholegrains, wholewheat bread, pasta, brown rice and pulses. Fruit and a handful of nuts and seeds can give you a natural energy boost throughout the day. It's also important that you eat your five portions of fresh fruits and vegetables; they are packed with the nutrients you need to beat fatigue. If you can tolerate dairy products, live yogurt might be helpful as it contains probiotics (beneficial bacteria) to keep your digestion healthy and fight *Candida albicans*. If you can't tolerate dairy products you might want to consider taking probiotics in supplement form. Ask at your chemist or consult a nutritionist for details.

Finally, take your time when eating your food. Don't shovel it down in seconds and then wonder why you feel so tired. Breaking down the food you eat demands a lot of energy from your body, so don't overload the system. Put your fork down between each bite. Take the time to really chew each mouthful. Give your stomach and digestive system a break.

B VITAMINS

The B vitamins are important if you are tired, as the deficiency symptoms of the major B vitamins is lack of energy. Make sure you are getting enough vitamin B in your diet and in your multivitamin.

CO-ENZYME Q10

Co-enzyme Q10, a substance present in all human tissue and organs, is a vital catalyst in the provision of energy for all our cells. It is a wonderful supplement for the heart and is routinely given to heart patients in Japan. There is as yet no conclusive proof that it can boost energy, but many experts believe that a consequence of a deficiency in co-enzyme Q10 is a reduction in energy.

COLOUR BOOST

Add red, orange or yellow to your surroundings to promote energy and confidence. Put flowers on your desk to give you a lift, or place brightly coloured accessories around your home to boost your spirits.

FLOWER POWER

You might like to try Bach Flower Remedies to help pep you up. Olive can help if you need an extra lift during a hard day's work, and hornbean can help if you find it hard to get up in the morning.

HERBAL HELP

Herbs can help energy levels. Fatigue following a long period of stress may be improved by taking diluted *Avena sativa* (wild oats) tincture. Take as directed until symptoms improve. Ginger can relieve flagging energy. Use it fresh in food or, for a quick pick-me-up, grate ginger into hot water and drink as a tea. Cinnamon could be added, as this spice also helps raise energy. Add clear honey to taste for a pleasant, warming, stimulating drink that also does wonders for the digestive system.

Perhaps one of the most well-known herbal remedies for boosting energy is ginseng. Research[6] shows that it can help restore vital energy and help the body to overcome stress, fatigue and weakness. Siberian ginseng is helpful as it works with your body's own needs, providing energy when required and helping to combat fatigue and stress when you are under pressure. It supports adrenal gland function and acts as a tonic to these glands. If you have been under mental or physical stress, Siberian ginseng can be extremely helpful and should be taken for about three months.

AROMATHERAPY

Aromatherapy oils such as basil and rosemary can be helpful for mental and physical fatigue. Try them in a vaporizer in your room, or add a few drops to your bath. Citrus fragrances such as grapefruit, lemon or orange are zesty and refreshing. You could also try burning 4 drops of balancing bergamot, 2 drops of relaxing cedarwood and 2 drops of energizing juniper essential oils for a refreshing lift.

HOMEOPATHY

The homeopathic remedy *Nux vomica* can alleviate low energy levels, poor sleeping patterns and tension headaches. If you feel mentally, emotionally and physically exhausted, try *Sepia*. Take one 30c potency dose daily for up to five days. *Kali phos* may alleviate burn-out after a period of intense activity such as exams or moving house. When the pressure is on, take a 6c potency tablet once a day for up to a week. Other remedies that are indicated for fatigue include: *Phosphoric acid*, *Picric acid*, *Arsenicum* and *China*.

YOGA

Yoga can help to realign your body, allowing vital energy to flow freely. Why not try a class and see if it works for you? Have a go now with the Half-moon stretch, which improves breathing and boosts energy:

Stand with your feet together, arms by your sides, breathing regularly. Inhale and bring your arms up, pressing the palms together. Exhale and bend slowly to one side, then hold the position for as long as you feel comfortable, breathing regularly. Inhale and return to the upright position. Then repeat on the other side.

EYE EXERCISES

If your eyes feel tired and heavy, close them and gently place your cupped palms over your eyesockets. Keep the palms in this position for a minute or so, gently pressing against the eye area while you breathe from your abdomen. If you work for long hours at VDU screens, or need to do a lot or reading or writing, it is important to remember to blink at regular intervals to lubricate your eyes and stop them feeling strained and dry.

NECK ROLLS

Loosing up your neck and shoulder muscles can also help, as these are the areas we often hold a lot of tension. Relax your jaw and drop your shoulders. Drop your head gently forward and slowly roll it round to your right shoulder, let the weight of your head take it back as far as it will go, then circle it towards your left shoulder. Breathe deeply and slowly and repeat, starting with the left shoulder. If you feel sluggish at work this will fully relax your head and neck muscles and give you a quick energy boost.

PUMP UP THE VOLUME

Music is wonderful for flagging spirits. Carry your favourite music in a portable player so you can get an instant energy-rush at the press of a button.

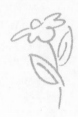

Week 3

At a Glance

DAY 1
Nutrition: Eat healthily, take your multivitamin and -mineral and make sure you get enough calcium and magnesium every day; do your PMS daily record and wall chart; eat more salads
Exercise: Exercise for 20 minutes and do your stretching
Emotional well-being: Positive thinking and PMS

DAY 2
Nutrition: Eat healthily, take your multivitamin and -mineral and make sure you get enough calcium and magnesium every day; do your PMS daily record and wall chart; sugar cravings and how to beat them
Exercise: 20 minutes and your stretching
Emotional well-being: Positive affirmations

DAY 3
Nutrition: Eat healthily, take your multivitamin and -mineral and

make sure you get enough calcium and magnesium every day; do your PMS daily record and wall chart

Exercise: 20 minutes, get some fresh air and plan a fun activity for the weekend

Emotional well-being: The Bubble

DAY 4

Nutrition: Eat healthily, take your multivitamin and -mineral and make sure you get enough calcium and magnesium every day; do your PMS daily record and wall chart; healthy snacking

Exercise: 20 minutes and your stretching routine

Emotional well-being: Being your own best friend

DAY 5

Nutrition: Eat healthily, take your multivitamin and -mineral and make sure you get enough calcium and magnesium every day; do your PMS daily record and wall chart; fibre and PMS

Exercise: 20 minutes and your stretching routine

Emotional well-being: Positive thinking

DAY 6

Nutrition: Eat healthily, take your multivitamin and -mineral and make sure you get enough calcium and magnesium every day; do your PMS daily record and wall chart; smoothies

Exercise: Have a day out and get lots of fresh air and exercise

Emotional well-being: Challenge your thinking

DAY 7

Nutrition: Eat healthily, take your multivitamin and -mineral and make sure you get enough calcium and magnesium every day; do your PMS daily record and wall chart; treat yourself and a loved one to a meal out

Exercise: Take the day off!

Emotional well-being: Making your own opportunities

VITALITY BOOSTER: Boosting your immune system

Day 1

NUTRITION

Sample Menu
Breakfast with multivitamin and -mineral, calcium and magnesium: Fruit salad
sprinkled with chopped nuts, slice of wholemeal toast with scraping of
butter, glass of diluted fresh-pressed apple juice
Snack: Low-fat digestive biscuit, glass of calcium-enriched skimmed milk
Lunch: Lean meat or fish, small jacket potato*, mushroom salad*, fresh
fruit, nuts, seeds
Snack: Small flapjack
Dinner: Pea and mushroom soup*, wholemeal roll with meat or fish and
salad, muesli bar with low-fat vanilla yogurt

Task for Today
Using the information from last week about raw foods, enzymes and
sprouts, aim to have a salad every day this week either as a main course
or as a side dish for lunch or dinner. If you have bought a juicer, make
sure you start using that, too. At the back of the book you'll find lots of
mouth-watering recipes for a variety of salads with some ideas for
dressings. You'll also find some fruit salad recipes and juice recipes.

EXERCISE
Do your 20-minute walk and gentle stretching routine. Remember, if this
is the day of your class or home video/home disco, you don't have to do
your walk as well.

EMOTIONAL WELL-BEING
Today we'd like you to consider some positive thinking and how it can
help ease your symptoms and boost your health and well-being. Studies[1]
show that people who are more optimistic about life feel healthier and
happier and women who think positively about themselves in their life
are more likely to do well in fighting PMS than those who feel that their
life is out of control.[2]

Negative feelings, like worry, fear and helplessness, all encourage the body to produce stress hormones, particularly cortisol, the hormone that can eat into your progesterone supply and create hormonal havoc, depression and fatigue. Positive thinking, on the other hand, will automatically boost your energy levels and improve your mood – and anything that can do that is bound to make you feel better.

Positive thinking is your always-available remedy for PMS. It really can improve your health and well-being. Don't believe us? Then have a go right now. Think about something that really makes you happy – your kids, your partner, your pet, your family, your holidays, your hobby or whatever brings magic, fun and love into your life. Think of a good joke. Think of the good things in your life. Think of beautiful and happy things. Chances are your breathing just deepened, your shoulders relaxed, and you're on your way to feeling better already.

Day 2

NUTRITION

Sample Menu
Breakfast with supplements: Half a grapefruit with low-fat yogurt, bowl of high-fibre breakfast cereal, glass of calcium-enriched skimmed or semi-skimmed milk
Snack: Fresh fruit with sesame seed crackers
Lunch: Egg and spinach cake* with green salad* and wholemeal bun; chopped bananas with low-fat custard
Snack: Low-fat wholemeal scone with clear honey
Dinner: Salmon dinner* with new potatoes and broccoli; baked apples with low-fat custard

Task for Today
Today we'd like you to think about the amount of sugar in your diet.

There have been times when I could quite literally have killed for a
chocolate bar. My partner is very long-suffering. He once drove 5 miles in
the middle of the night to get me my chocolate fix. It sounds crazy but I get
such powerful cravings. **Katy, 25**

It can be so hard to choose a salad or piece of fruit when all you really
want is to sink your teeth into a mouth-watering bar of chocolate! We are
not going to pretend that raw food has the same satisfaction factor as
chocolate, sweets and biscuits. (Raw foods, fruits and vegetables can taste
delicious and satisfying, but it takes time for your taste buds to adapt if
you are used to sugar.) Instead we are going to explain to you why too
much sugar in your diet can make your symptoms worse. Hopefully this
will be enough to convince you to keep sweet food choices to a minimum,
especially in the week or so before your period.

Studies[3] show that women with PMS do crave sugary foods more than
women without, and that the higher the sugar content of a woman's diet,
the more severe her symptoms. This is because during the week before
your period your body becomes extra-responsive to insulin, the hormone
that sends glucose to the cells where it is used for energy. But the insulin
clears away too much glucose, leaving you with low blood sugar and
cravings for sweet food. So what do you do? You reach for a bar of
chocolate. Trouble is, this makes the situation even worse.

Eating sugar triggers the release of more insulin, the same hormone that
is making you crave sugar in the first place. Sugar interferes with the
efficient processing of oestrogen in the liver. Oestrogen levels rise and you
end up feeling tired, moody and hungry again. Sugar overload also
activates the adrenal glands to release adrenaline, which pushes blood
sugar levels up but increases anxiety. Adrenaline stimulates the release of
cortisol, which not only causes sugar cravings but makes it harder for
your body to use progesterone effectively. And if that weren't enough,
sugar depletes the body of essential nutrients, creating deficiencies which
can bring on symptoms of PMS.

Sugar-rich snacks or drinks do give you a quick energy boost, but a slump will always follow, leaving you craving even more sugar, especially chocolate. This is hardly surprising, as chocolate contains magnesium and an amino acid that can ease depression. But unfortunately a high-sugar food like chocolate is the last thing you should be eating right now. It's a vicious cycle of short highs and long lows.

So how can you stop yourself turning into a sugar demon? Here are some tips to think about today; we'll be reinforcing them throughout the plan.

- Do your best to avoid sugar and sugary food in the week or so before your period. Foods such as breakfast cereals, cakes, biscuits, ice cream, jam, pudding and all refined foods like white bread and rice (they act like sugar because of their lack of fibre).
- Whenever you get that sugar craving, try to eat complex carbohydrates like wholegrain breads, cereal or pasta along with a little protein like low-fat cottage cheese or skimmed milk.
- Remember that fruits contain natural sugars that can drive blood sugars up, so try to eat fruits and vegetables in conjunction with a small amount of protein, such as a handful of nuts and seeds.
- Sugar hides in lots of foods, so always check the sugar content of the food you eat. Don't forget that sugar has lots of different names, including: brown sugar, concentrated fruit juice, corn syrup, dextrose, fructose, glucose, honey, lactose, maltose, molasses, raw sugar and sucrose. If you see any of the above listed as one of the first four ingredients on the label, that means sugar is one of the main ingredients. Avoid it because it is a high-sugar food.
- Get rid of your sugar bowl.
- Get the low-sugar versions of jams, canned fruit, jellies and juices.
- Buy vanilla wafers, gingersnaps or low-fat digestives if you can't live without biscuits.
- Try adding cinnamon, ginger, nutmeg and other spices to food for a sweet taste without sugar. Make sure you eat little and often. Leaving long gaps between meals means blood sugar levels will drop again and you may find yourself reaching for a quick boost to perk you up.
- Alcohol and caffeine can make sugar cravings worse. If you can't avoid

them altogether it is best to have them in moderation. A few glasses of wine a week, not every day. A cup of coffee or two a day, not every hour. A small bar of chocolate, not a family-sized one.

• Foods that contain artificial sweeteners should be avoided or kept to a minimum. They often contain chemicals such as aspartame, which have been linked to mood swings and depression.

Starting today, gradually cut down your sugar intake. You may think we are asking too much by suggesting that you cut down on sugar, especially at the time of the month when you would kill for it. It may seem daunting right now, but you'll be surprised how your taste buds will adapt and it won't be long before sweet, refined foods start to taste overly sweet and you prefer the taste of healthier alternatives. You'll also find that your cravings start to disappear once you start to eat healthily according the 12-week plan guidelines.

I can't believe that I used to eat so much sugar. At the height of my PMS I was eating several chocolate bars a day as well as sugary, carbonated sweets and drinks. Not to mention the sugar I heaped in my tea and coffee and on my cereal in the morning. I went to see a nutritionist when my PMS – along with my weight – started to get out of hand. I felt awful when she told me I was eating enough sugar for five or six people every day. The first week was tough (my taste buds craved sweetness) but by the second week I was making progress – two teaspoons of sugar in my tea instead of four and a couple of chocolate bars a week, not every day. Then a few weeks more of healthy eating and I started to find the thought of all that sugar quite unpleasant. Cutting back on sugar really helped me. Not only did the weight start to drop off but my mood was better, I had more energy and, best of all, I had my first PMS-free month. **Lynn, 39**

EXERCISE

Do your 20-minute walk and gentle stretching, and book in time at the weekend for a much longer walk around a local beauty spot or local park. Plan to walk somewhere where the scenery is beautiful, even if it means travelling or having a whole day out. The fresh air will be energizing and you'll also get your exercise. You may even get more of a strenuous workout if there is an odd hill or two to climb. Think about whether you would like to bring a picnic or have a pub or café lunch. You might like to ask your partner or a friend to come with you, or you may prefer to spend the time alone.

Spending time in green spaces boosts oxygen intake, the feel-good factor and your mental health. Trees and green plants give out lots of energizing oxygen. All you need to do for a quick energy- and mood-boost is to go for a brisk walk and breathe it in.

EMOTIONAL WELL-BEING

Studies show[4] that when women with PMS feel good about themselves, they feel happier, and when they feel happier, symptoms ease. When they feel bad about themselves, their health suffers. So today we'd like you to consider the way you think and the way you talk about yourself.

Do you say things like:

I'm no good.
It's only me.
I wouldn't be any good at that.
I can't.
Trust me to mess things up.

If you talk negatively about yourself all the time, it won't be long before you start agreeing with yourself. Today we'd like you to stop and reflect whenever you put yourself down, and instead of the usual negative we'd like you to say something positive. Replace 'I can't' with 'I'll try' or 'I'll do my best.' Replace 'I'm no good' with 'I learn from my mistakes.' Replace 'I'm useless' with 'I can learn.' Replace 'It's only me' with 'It's me and I'm a terrific person.' Even if you don't feel like you can really believe this right now, try it.

When you say positive things to yourself you are retraining your mind. It's rather like learning a new language. The words and phrases come before the understanding. It's a struggle at first, but then you start to see the bigger picture. Believing the positive things you say about yourself will eventually come. For now, just keep telling yourself positive things over and over again. Start reprogramming your mind.

If you feel low it may feel impossible even to say, let alone believe, that you are special, lovable and important. But it is at these times that you most need positive thinking. Belief is very strong medicine. When it feels impossible to be positive, keep practising and tell yourself positive things. Practise saying that you are wonderful, creative, happy, deserving and significant – because you are.

It may help to create a list of positive affirmations. Keep these affirmations in the present tense, keep them positive, and practise saying them all the time. Refer to your list as soon as you feel low. Use some of our examples below or create your own:

I value myself.
I am a wonderfully creative person.
I deserve to be happy.
I can handle challenges.

Day 3

NUTRITION

Sample Menu
Breakfast with supplements: Cereal with a piece of chopped fruit, sprinkled with nuts and raisins with low-fat milk or yogurt, glass of fresh-pressed diluted apple juice
Snack: Fresh fruit with handful of unsalted nuts
Lunch: Tofu and mushroom kebab* with wholemeal rice and salad; apple crunch*
Snack: Sesame biscuits and a glass of soya, nut or skimmed organic milk
Dinner: Home-made soup and mixed bean salad*, slice of low-fat apple and cinnamon cake

Task for Today

Today we'd like to focus on fibre and how it can help you beat PMS.

Fibre is the term used to refer to the part of plants that your body cannot digest. It can wash away wastes and toxins and speed up the amount of time it takes for food to pass through your intestines. It can also act like a sponge and prevent substances your body doesn't need any more, such as excess cholesterol and oestrogen, from being reabsorbed into your body.

Fibre is important if you have PMS because it slows down the conversion of carbohydrates into blood sugar, thus helping to maintain blood sugar balance. Fibre also ensures that digestion is healthy, fat absorption is controlled, toxins are removed from the body, energy is released, stools are well formed and waste can pass through at a steady rate, preventing the build-up of hormones and toxins in the gut where they can be reabsorbed into the bloodstream. An adequate fibre intake also ensures that you get that full-up feeling after you have eaten. For all these reasons, if you don't eat enough fibre, PMS symptoms are likely to get worse.

Fibre is divided into two different types: soluble, which means it can dissolve in water, and insoluble, meaning it won't. Insoluble fibre is found in wheat bran, green leafy vegetables and the skins of fruits and root vegetables. It bulks up the stool, absorbs water and stimulates the contraction of the intestinal walls so waste is pushed through faster. Insoluble fibre helps prevent diabetes, colon cancer and heart disease. Sources of soluble fibre include oats, beans, parley, psyllium seeds and many vegetables and fruit. This type of fibre slows down glucose absorption after a meal, keeping your blood sugar levels on an even keel. Soluble fibre also helps lower cholesterol.

Research supports the idea of eating a high-fibre diet if you have blood sugar problems. Dr James Anderson at the University of Kentucky showed that diabetes control is greatly enhanced when 40 to 50g of carbohydrate is eaten a day. A study in the *Lancet* showed that the blood sugar levels of people with diabetes who regularly ate fibre from legumes, such as beans and peas, significantly improved. Many women with PMS have trouble with blood sugar levels, so a high-fibre diet makes sense.

> For five years PMS virtually took over my life. I'd plan meetings, social events, holidays around it. Then after my third child I decided to go on a diet. I went to a nutritionist and learned about eating more fibre to give you that full-up feeling and make sure food passes through quickly. The first week of my new healthy eating plan was a joke. I spent most of it on the toilet. I thought 'This can't be right' and phoned my doctor. He said that it was just my digestive system getting used to a new way of eating and it wouldn't take long before things settled down. He was right: within two weeks it did and within six weeks not only had I lost 7 pounds but my PMS symptoms started to clear up, too. **Susan, 36**

If you are not used to eating a high-fibre diet you need to introduce more fibre into your diet slowly to give your bowels time to adapt. Make sure you drink at least eight glasses of water a day. Fibre draws water, so you need to drink a lot to process it properly. Don't be surprised if your stools look more bulky the more fibre you eat. Ideally you should aim to eat between 20 and 30 grams of fibre a day – any more than that and you might be pushing your system too hard. If you make sure you eat at least five fruits and veg a day, and six to ten servings of wholemeal grains a day, you should be eating enough fibre – but if you eat a lot of refined foods you may not be getting enough.

It's best to stay away from fibre supplements or laxatives. You won't get the nutrients or the full-up feeling you get from fibre-rich foods. Real food is your best source of fibre. Always choose wholegrains over refined foods and remember that the closer a plant food is to its natural state, the more fibre it is likely to have. Bran breakfast cereals offer a lot of fibre, but don't rely on this totally for your fibre intake. Try to distribute your fibre intake throughout the day.

EXERCISE
Do your 20-minute walk and stretching routine. Don't forget if the weather is horrible you can still dance at home to your favourite music.

EMOTIONAL WELL-BEING

Today we'd like you to find the positive in negative situations. We'd like you to cancel out the negative thoughts. For example, if you have an argument with a loved one, don't focus on that – think about the fun times you have had. If work is driving you crazy, think about what you are planning to do at the weekend. If a relationship ends, focus your attention on the new possibilities that lie ahead. The positive is always there – today we'd like you to leave negative thoughts backstage and bring the positive ones into the limelight.

We'd also like you to try this exercise to protect yourself from negativity from both yourself and others:

The Bubble

Close your eyes and relax. Become aware of your breathing. Concentrate on breathing in and out and shut out the sounds going on outside. When you feel relaxed, imagine that a beautiful bubble is floating down in front of you rather like the ones you often see kids blowing at parties. Look at it slowly settle on the floor in front of you and see how beautifully the bubble reflects the light. Now watch your bubble start to grow, bigger and bigger until it is twice the size you are. Now reach forward and touch the bubble, pushing your hand and then the rest of your body through so you are standing inside. Watch as a ray of light surrounds and seals the bubble. You feel safe and protected inside. No one but you can step inside. Nothing and no one can harm you.

Whenever you feel low or threatened by others, use this exercise. Visualize your bubble and step quickly into it. You will feel protected and safe.

Day 4

NUTRITION

Sample Menu
Breakfast with supplements: Half a grapefruit, 1 boiled egg, slice wholemeal toast with a scraping of butter, glass of calcium-enriched skimmed or semi-skimmed milk
Snack: Fresh fruit and handful of nuts
Lunch: Pasta salad*; fruit kebab* with vegetables
Snack: Oatcakes with low-fat spread or cottage cheese
Dinner: Grilled chicken, fish or tofu and big green salad with lemon juice and hemp/pumpkin seed oil dressing; banana surprise*

Task for Today
Re-read the information on Day 2 about sugar cravings. Prepare a couple of healthy, nutritious snacks and put them in the fridge, or take them with you to work or in the car so that if hunger strikes you have them at hand and you won't be tempted to dash into the nearest shop for chocolate, biscuits, cakes or crisps. Here's a list of healthy snacks:

- Vegetable sticks
- 3 fresh dates
- 4 fresh apricots
- 1 apple
- 1 pear
- 1 plum
- 1 jaffa cake
- 1 small flapjack
- 1 fig roll
- 1 low-fat granola, muesli or fruit bar
- 1 low-fat scone/muffin
- Breadsticks with vegetable dips
- Low-fat cottage cheese with a cracker
- 2 Ryvita (rye crackers) with Marmite
- Small bag of unsalted or sweetened popcorn

- Small bag of twiglets
- 2 rice cakes with unsalted butter
- Frozen fruit lollies
- Low-fat yogurt with handful of nuts
- Sesame seed crackers

EXERCISE
Do your 20-minute walk and stretching routine.

EMOTIONAL WELL-BEING
Once again today we'd like you to watch your language. How do you talk to yourself? Are you kind and considerate or are you harsh and judgemental? If your best friend called you and wanted reassurance, would you use negative words and tell her she was no good? No, you would offer comfort and support. Why not do the same for yourself?

When things get tough, become your own best friend. Imagine that you have stepped outside of your body and that you are standing by yourself. Now hold your hand. What would you say that was reassuring and comforting? How would you help this person feel better? What would you say? Would you tell her that she is doing well and that she has lots of good qualities and that good things do lie ahead? Talk to yourself the way you would to a best friend or loved one who was feeling down.

This technique is really great when negative thoughts start to overwhelm you. It's simple and effective.

Day 5

NUTRITION

Sample Menu
Breakfast with supplements: Skimmed or soya milk porridge with small banana and chopped nuts plus a glass of fresh-pressed apple juice
Snack: Celery and carrot sticks

Lunch: Couscous soup* with wholegrain roll and lentil salad; low-fat yogurt and fresh fruit
Snack: Low-fat cheese scone with scraping of butter
Dinner: Mixed bean and vegetable casserole with brown rice*; bowl of raspberries sprinkled with cashews and a low-fat yogurt topping

Task for Today
Re- read the information on Day 3 about fibre and make a real effort to include enough fibre in your meals.

EXERCISE
Do your 20-minute walk and stretching routine.

EMOTIONAL WELL-BEING
Re-read the positive-thinking information and exercises in Days 1 to 4, above. Now try to do the exercises throughout the day so you get lots of positive-thinking boosts. Record how you feel in your emotional diary. Here are a few other exercises you might like to try over the next few weeks:

Getting Rid of Guilt
Women often try to be everything to everybody, and end up feeling more and more exhausted. If this is you stop, for a moment. Tell yourself that you always do your best and imagine guilty feelings floating away like a balloon. Let your balloon go and never think about it again.

Focusing On Your Strengths
When you feel low, lift yourself up by focusing on your strengths. Write down as many as you can think of. Be proud of yourself. Self-respect opens the door to optimism.

Creating Success for Yourself
Find a comfortable place, close your eyes and relax. Follow your breathing and then see your success in action. Picture the scene

that you would like to create. See yourself being successful, happy and positive about life. You look confident and relaxed. Feel what it is like to be a success. See people treating you with the respect you deserve. Make this vision as real as you can. See and hear the whole thing in colour, create the sound effects, feel the reality of your success. When you are ready, let your thoughts return, open your eyes and come back to the room.

Stop Comparing Yourself with Others
Do you ever feel that you are not as good, clever, lovely as someone else? Each time you compare yourself with other people, you are mistrusting yourself. The next time you find yourself comparing, tell yourself that you are unique. Accept and make the most of your differences. They are what makes you a unique and original person with your own special place in the world.

Day 6

NUTRITION

Sample Menu
Breakfast with supplements: Fruit salad sprinkled with nuts, slice of wholegrain bread plus scraping of butter and jam, glass of calcium-enriched skimmed milk
Snack: Low-fat cottage cheese and cracker
Lunch: Cheese and broccoli soup* plus wholegrain roll and scraping of butter; nut roast*
Snack: Low-fat yogurt topped with fresh fruit
Dinner: Tuna fish cakes*, broccoli and vegetable rice; baked peach filled with a tablespoon of low-fat soft cheese mixed with one large amaretti biscuit crushed and a drop of vanilla essence.

Task for Today
Today we would like you to treat yourself to a smoothie.

Not only do smoothies taste comforting and delicious, they have the added bonus of being rich in vitamins, minerals and fibre – and you know how important these are if you have PMS. Smoothies are made in a blender rather than a juicer, which is particularly good for liquefying bananas. You can put bananas through your juicer but they need to be very soft and to be followed by very watery fruits, like melons.

You can make lots of wonderful drinks in a blender. We've listed a few recipes in Appendix 4 for you to try, but part of the fun of using a blender is creating your own delicious smoothies. Make sure you remove all the skin and pips/stones before placing a fruit in your blender. Smoothies are especially good when blended with low-fat yogurt or calcium-enriched soymilk, which gives them the texture of milk shakes or melted ice-cream without the fat or sugar.

EXERCISE

Have your day out as planned. On your day out you don't need to do your walk or stretches. On the day you are not going out, increase your walking time to 30 minutes.

Last week we talked about the magical 20-minute mark when you exercise. We'd now like to take that one stage further and explain to you why any exercise you do that is over 20 minutes will be of even greater benefit. This is because at around the 20-minute mark you switch from burning mainly carbohydrate to burning mainly fat. Exercise that is over the 20-minute mark burns off fat, speeds up your metabolism and helps balance your hormones, thus easing symptoms of PMS. And the effects last way beyond your workout. Studies show that fit people burn more calories than unfit people do even when they are resting. So the more you exercise, the more your muscles build up and the more efficient your metabolism gets at counter-acting the effects of blood sugar imbalance which can trigger PMS.

EMOTIONAL WELL-BEING

When you are premenstrual, feelings seem out of control – but research shows that it is your thoughts that determine your feelings. If you can get a grip on your thoughts, this can lead to a change in the way you feel. So today we are going to look at five ways you can manage difficult feelings, such as sadness, anger and guilt.

1. Don't believe everything you feel
Just because you feel something does not mean it is true. For example, PMS can make you feel terrible, but this does not mean you are terrible. You are the one in charge of your feelings, not the other way round.

2. Stop exaggerating
PMS is likely to make you take the negative in a situation and blow it up out of all proportion. One argument with your partner is grounds for divorce. One setback at work makes you question your ability to do your job. The kids are a little difficult and you feel you are a failure as a mother. The negative potential is all that you see.

Try to combat exaggerating. Stop using words like 'terrible', 'disaster' and 'horrendous'. Since you are stuck in a negative rut you have to make a real effort to look for balance. Focusing on just the negative is unrealistic and unfair. Yes, you had an argument with your partner, but most of the time you get on really well. Yes, you had a problem at work, but this doesn't mean you can't do your job. Yes, the kids can be a nightmare sometimes and you lose your temper, but most of the time you are a great mum.

3. Don't take it personally
When you have PMS the world tends to shrink. Everything seems to revolve around you and the way you feel. Something goes wrong and it's your fault. Your partner works late and it is because he wants to get away from you.

Stop thinking that everything revolves around you. Lots of things have nothing to do with you. People have other things going on in their lives apart from you.

4. Stop blaming
Other people can't 'make' you feel in a certain way. For example, your

partner asks you to do something and you become angry because you think he should know how tired you are. But it is your responsibility to tell other people what is going through your mind. Other people are not mind-readers.

5. Fortune-telling

When you feel low and see only the negative, the future looks bleak. But how do you know things aren't going to work out? You are not a fortune-teller. Things may turn out bad, but they may also turn out well. Look at things with some perspective and get rid of over-the-top pessimism.

Becoming aware of how your thoughts affect your feelings is a big step forward. The next time you feel low, pay attention to your thinking patterns. You don't need to replace negative thoughts with positive ones all the time. You just need to replace them with more realistic, balanced ones. But fortunately a realistic outlook is often much more optimistic than a negative one. Realistic thoughts take into account both the negative and the positive, but negative thoughts just focus on the negative. So today when negative thoughts appear, don't treat them as facts because you are thinking them. Most of the time they are inaccurate, misleading and unrealistic. Every time you get a negative thought, challenge it rationally and replace it with more realistic, constructive thoughts.

Day 7

NUTRITION

Sample Menu
Breakfast with supplements: Slice of wholegrain toast with a teaspoon of peanut butter, small banana, fresh-pressed juice
Snack: Bowl of cherries and a handful of nuts, glass of calcium-enriched soymilk
Lunch: Large bowl of vegetable soup* and lean turkey or low-fat cheese salad sandwich

Snack: Apple and one jaffa cake or low-fat chocolate biscuit/cookie
Dinner: Treat yourself and your partner or a friend to a meal out

Healthy eating does not mean you can't eat out anymore. You just need to pay a little more attention to the food you are ordering. Here are some helpful tips:

- Don't eat from the bread basket.
- Drink water or fruit juice rather than alcohol or fizzy, sweet drinks.
- Try vegetable soup or clear soup for starters.
- Always ask for vegetables instead of chips.
- Have a side salad with your main course.
- Go for tomato- or wine-based sauces rather than cheesy, buttery ones.
- Ask for dressings to be on the side so you can dress your food/salad yourself.
- Have a fruit-based dessert.
- If you like to eat Chinese or Indian food, ask for plain boiled rice rather than fried – and again, watch those sauces.
- Choose grilled fishes or meat rather than fried.
- Fresh fish dishes, simple stuffed vegetable dishes or large salads are a good choice if you enjoy Mediterranean food.
- If you like Mexican, stick to the salsa, fresh and steamed vegetables and grilled meat and skip the tortilla chips and cheese.
- Don't be afraid to ask for food that isn't on the menu, or for an ingredient you know isn't good for you, to be left out of the dish.
- If your plate is very full, eat only half of it and ask the waiter to bag the rest up for you to take home.
- If dinner is going to be late, eat a balanced snack – for example a piece of fruit and a handful of nuts – when you would normally eat dinner so you won't be tempted to eat too much when you do go out.

Task for Today

Make a list of restaurants and take-aways in your local area where you can order healthy options.

EXERCISE

Take it easy today. You don't need to do your 20 minutes of exercise, but do keep as active as you can throughout the day.

EMOTIONAL WELL-BEING

Studies[5] show that people who feel grateful for their blessings feel better able to cope with difficulties. The tendency is always to think about what we have not got. A better approach is to appreciate and value what we have already.

Write out a list of all the blessings in your life and keep it in a place where you can read it often. If you find it hard to think about how lucky you are, then today we'd like you to start bringing more blessings into your life. Remember the happier and more fulfilled you are, the easier it will be for you to beat PMS.

VITALITY BOOSTER

Your Immune System

Why is boosting your immune system important if you have PMS? Because colds and niggling health problems can sap your energy, make you feel more negative and make your body use up valuable energy and nutrients that you need to beat PMS.

Your immune system is your basic defence against infection and toxins from the environment. Learning how to support your immune system and your body's own defence system is crucial for good health, vitality and for beating PMS.

To eat right for your immune system, make sure that your diet includes enough of the antioxidant vitamins: A, C and E. These vitamins are thought to protect against a variety of illnesses, from minor infections like colds to major diseases like cancer. They are also thought to fight the damaging effect of free radicals.

Free radicals are created when oxygen is converted into energy. To imagine the process, think of a car rusting or an apple going brown after it is cut in half. A similar process occurs in your body. A certain number of free radicals are required in our bodies to kill bacteria, but in excess they can damage cell membranes and encourage the development of disease. Antioxidant nutrients fight the process of oxidation that occurs non-stop in our bodies.

Since they have such an important function, let's consider them in turn:

BETACAROTENE

Betacarotene is converted to vitamin A when it is in your body. It can neutralize the ageing effects of sunlight on the skin. Yellow or orange fruits and vegetables such as carrots and mangos, sweet potatoes, spinach, watercress, tomatoes, asparagus, broccoli and peaches are rich in betacarotene. Ideally you should aim for five portions of betacarotene-rich foods daily.

VITAMIN C

Vitamin C plays a significant role in supporting the immune system and fighting off infection. It is found in most fresh fruits and vegetables. Good food sources include the following: blackcurrants, parsley, raw greenpeppers, strawberries, watercress, sprouts, lemons, oranges, broccoli, grapefruit and cauliflower. Your body needs a constant daily supply of vitamin C, so eat as many vitamin C-rich foods as you can every day.

VITAMIN E

Vitamin E has been hailed as one of the most important antioxidant nutrients because of the way it can strengthen white blood cells against infection. It works in tandem with vitamin C, so you need to make sure you have optimum quantities of both vitamins in your diet. Vitamin E is obtained mainly from vegetables oils, nuts and whole grains. Make sure you eat vitamin E foods daily.

POSITIVE THINKING

The next way to boost your immune system we've already discussed this week: positive thinking. Your state of mind has a profound effect on your health and well-being. Don't you always get a cold when you are under stress or feeling down? A recent study at the University of Reading showed that those who recalled happy memories had elevated immune antibodies in their saliva, whereas those who remembered unhappy things had depressed antibodies. Studies of this kind show that we need to have positive thoughts and feelings supplied on a regular basis to give our immune system a constant, daily boost.

Sensual pleasure also plays a part in boosting immunity, according to research at the University of Westminster. Subjects were asked to smell a wide variety of pleasant and unpleasant odours, then their saliva was measured for immune antibody levels. Attractive odours boosted levels, while unpleasant ones suppressed them. Studies like this show you just how important it is to seek out positive, uplifting and pleasurable experiences.

EXERCISE

Exercise helps the immune system by conditioning the lymphatic system. It is the function of the lymphatic system to filter out any impurities before they are channelled into the bloodstream. For the essential process of detoxification the lymphatic system depends on the muscle pressure that occurs every time you move or exercise.

Regular exercise is the best way to stimulate the lymphatic system, but other techniques such as massage, bathing, hydrotherapy or dry skin brushing may also have benefits. For dry skin brushing all you need is a natural bristle brush to brush your skin before showering or bathing. The brush should be used in large sweeping movements which cover your body moving in a downward direction towards your trunk and upwards from your feet, legs and hips.

ALTERNATIVE REMEDIES

As we've stressed, the best way to deal with minor infections is to concentrate on ways to boost your immune system so it can fight illness effectively. If you do fall ill, however, alternative home remedies can support you through times of illness, leaving you less prone to complications. Below we've listed a few natural remedies that may be an excellent alternative to antibiotics (which can do as much harm as good to your immune system) for minor problems such as cystitis, sore throats, coughs or thrush. Follow the instructions enclosed with the remedies themselves, but if symptoms persist or are severe seek professional help immediately.

Problem	Blocked sinuses
Solution	If your sinuses feel blocked, use a humidifier or place bowls of cold water near a radiator to humidify the atmosphere. You might also like to add a few drops of lavender, tea tree or peppermint essential oils to a steam inhalation to clear a stuffy nose.
Problem	Colds, flu, viral infection
Solution	Echinacea can help your body fight viral infections such as flu, colds and blocked sinuses. You can take it in tablet form or tincture form. Take as long as the infection lasts.

Elderberry extract may be able to limit the spread of a virus and stimulate recovery from flu or chest infections within three days. Take in lozenge or liquid form.

An infusion of basil with a pinch of cloves taken when you have a cold can feel comforting, and also encourages you to sweat.

Herbalist Jenny Jones from the Creative Health Centre in Leamington Spa, Warwickshire, says yarrow breaks a fever, elderflower alleviates catarrh, and peppermint is cooling and calming.

Boneset is a North American herb and a good immune system-booster for a woman who has had flu for a while and is trying to shake it off.

Oscillococcinum is a homeopathic remedy often used to treat patients suffering from cold or flu. Take in tablet form according to the instructions of a homeopathic pharmacy. Other homeopathic remedies used for colds and flu include

Belladonna, Gelsemium, Nat mur and Pulsatilla. Ask a homeopathic pharmacist for details.

Eat garlic to ward off infection (raw if you can as its fresher than capsules) and take plenty of vitamin C.

Problem	Sore throat
Solution	Antibiotics will be offered for infections such as tonsillitis, but natural remedies can help. Sipping warm infusions of water with a dash of lemon and teaspoonful of honey may soothe a sore throat. You could also gargle with a teaspoonful of salt and vinegar in a cup of warm water – be careful not to swallow.

Grapefruit seed extract is thought to have antibiotic properties and is especially recommended for throat infection. It comes in tablet or liquid form and should be taken as long as symptoms persist. You might also like to try licorice.

If the soreness seems to be signalling the start of a cold the homeopathic remedy Aconite can stop it progressing further. Propolis is made by bees to protect the hives from infection and invasion, and it soothes pain. Also gargling with a few drops of tea tree oil or a pinch of salt in a glass of warm water can also help.

Problem	Coughs
Solution	Some coughs linger long after colds and flu have gone. Trudy Norris, herbalist and president of the National Institute of Medical Herbalists, suggests an infusion of thyme, which is antiseptic, clears phlegm and fights chest infections. Put a heaped tablespoonful of dried thyme into a litre of boiling water. Add a teaspoonful of honey to relieve irritation. Sipping a mixture of a teaspoonful of honey and warm water can help prevent persistent coughing at night.
Problem	Stress
Solution	Yoga and tai chi are good for calming the mind. St John's Wort can ease depression, and valerian aids sleep. Homeopathic Gelsemium and the Bach Flower remedy white chestnut soothe an overactive mind.

Problem   Cystitis

Solution   Drink plenty of water and try mild herbal teas such as
camomile and dandelion. Avoid tea, coffee or alcohol.

Cranberry has a reputation for reducing the incidence of
urinary tract infections. You need to drink lots of water, too. If
you have a history of cystitis, a glass of cranberry juice a day
may discourage infection. Make sure you find the
unsweetened kind, and dilute it with water or another fruit
juice to make it tasty.

Herbal remedies uva ursi and echinacea help too. Tea tree
oil can also protect against a range of viral, bacterial and
fungal infections. It should not be taken internally but used
as an external treatment in baths to soothe athlete's foot or
to ease symptoms of thrush and cystitis.

Problem   Digestive problems

Solution   If acidity and general digestive discomfort follow eating a
heavy meal, try sipping a soothing drink made from
powdered slippery elm and warm milk.

Discomfort and flatulence may respond well to an
infusion of fennel, peppermint or lemon balm.

Sucking a piece of crystallized ginger or drinking ginger
tea may also settle the stomach.

Aloe vera is thought to be a powerful antiseptic and
enhancer of the immune system. It is especially useful for
stomach upsets. It can be taken in the form of juice or tablets
for internal use, or in the form of gel as an antiseptic or
soothing agent for burns.

A gripey stomach responds well to ginger, while
peppermint is good for several digestive problems. Cut up
about 1 inch of ginger root, infuse it in a pan of boiling water
and drink it as a tea to calm bloating and pain. Just a sniff of
peppermint oil can relieve queasy stomachs. Peppermint oil
tablets are an effective remedy for all kinds of stomach
problems.

After too much alcohol, milk thistle detoxifies the liver,
while the homeopathic remedy Nux vom is good if you have

overindulged in food or drink, if you are getting feelings of
sickness, or to help you recover after a stomach upset.

Problem   Back pain

Solution   Regular yoga and toning can strengthen your back and ease
muscle tension.

Instead of anti-inflammatory drugs, which have side-
effects, there are several herbs which provide pain relief.
White willow contains aspirin-like constituents but, unlike
aspirin, is kind to the stomach. Devil's claw and bromelain
(pineapple) extract are both natural anti-inflammatories.

Problem   Cold sores

Solution   Licorice is thought to act as a tonic for the immune system
after it has been suppressed by a period of stress. It may help
your body fight throat infection, thrush and cold sores. Take
in capsule form as long as symptoms appear.

Problem   Headaches

Solution   Apply cold compresses to the spot where the pain is
radiating. This helps relieve headaches by constricting blood
vessels and easing muscle spasms. Leave a damp cloth in the
freezer for 10 minutes or use a cold gelpack.

A salve made from ginger, peppermint oils and winter
green oil rubbed on the nape of the neck and temples can
help relieve tension headaches. For sinus headaches, rub the
salve across the sinus area.

Ginkgo biloba improves circulation to the brain and may
be helpful.

Other herbs that may relieve headache pain include mint,
rosemary, burdock root, fenugreek and lavender.

GENERAL GUIDELINES WHEN FIGHTING INFECTION

- When infection strikes you should keep your fluid intake high at all
times but especially if you have a fever or an infection, in order to
flush toxins out of the body. Choose mineral water, herbal teas and
fruit juices, and avoid black tea and coffee, which can act as diuretics,
increasing the amount of liquid that is excreted from your body.

- Keep your meals light and avoid heavy or fatty foods that take a long time to be digested and use up energy needed to fight infection.
- Make sure that you are getting enough vitamin C, enough rest and enough time out.
- You might also like to think about including garlic regularly in your diet to discourage the development of recurrent infections. Garlic is thought to be an antibiotic and nourisher of the immune system. Although you can eat garlic in your diet it is difficult to include the amounts you need to have a therapeutic effect and still keep up an active social life! You can instead opt for one-a-day garlic tablets.

Week 4

At a Glance

DAY 1
Nutrition: Eat healthily, take your multivitamin and -mineral and make sure you get enough calcium and magnesium every day; do your PMS daily record and wall chart; essential fatty acids – Omega-3
Exercise: Take the day off!
Emotional well-being: Coping with PMS anger and mood swings

DAY 2
Nutrition: Eat healthily, take your multivitamin and -mineral and make sure you get enough calcium and magnesium every day; do your PMS daily record and wall chart; essential fatty acids – Omega-6
Exercise: Do your 30-minute walk, your stretching and check our your local swimming pool
Emotional well-being: Asking for support from those around you

DAY 3

Nutrition: Eat healthily, take your multivitamin and -mineral and make sure you get enough calcium and magnesium every day; do your PMS daily record and wall chart; fats that harm and fats that heal

Exercise: Do your 30 minutes of exercise, your stretching and think about joining some dance classes

Emotional well-being: RETHINK

DAY 4

Nutrition: Eat healthily, take your multivitamin and -mineral and make sure you get enough calcium and magnesium every day; do your PMS daily record and wall chart; check out your local health food store

Exercise: 30 minutes of exercise, your stretching routine, try some abdominals

Emotional well-being: Coping when the tension mounts

DAY 5

Nutrition: Eat healthily, take your multivitamin and -mineral and make sure you get enough calcium and magnesium every day; do your PMS daily record and wall chart; include nuts and seeds with every meal

Exercise: 30 minutes of exercise plus stretching and abdominal work

Emotional well-being: Quick 'in control' strategies

DAY 6

Nutrition: Eat healthily, take your multivitamin and -mineral and make sure you get enough calcium and magnesium every day; do your PMS daily record and wall chart; re-read this week's info, do a shopping list and plan next week's meals

Exercise: 30 minutes of exercise, plus stretching and abdominal work

Emotional well-being: The importance of expressing how you feel

> **DAY 7**
> *Nutrition*: Eat healthily, take your multivitamin and -mineral and get enough calcium and magnesium every day; do your PMS daily record and wall chart
> *Exercise*: 30 minutes of exercise and stretching, check your posture
> *Emotional well-being*: The importance of correct breathing
> *VITALITY BOOSTER*: Having more fun

Day 1

NUTRITION

Sample Menu
Breakfast with supplements: Bran muffin, low-fat yogurt, glass of fresh-pressed apple juice
Snack: Slice of banana and walnut cake, glass of calcium-enriched skimmed or semi-skimmed milk
Lunch: Vegetable stew*; fresh fruit
Snack: Handful of mixed seeds and an apple
Dinner: Tuna pasta* with mixed salad; rice dessert with nutmeg

Task for Today
Exploring essential fatty acids.

Review the information on essential fatty acids on pages 21–2. Remember that saturated fats are not good for you and that eating them can lead to poor health, while essential fatty acids (EFAs) – found in nuts, seeds and oily fish – are needed by every human cell. They balance hormones, insulate nerve cells and keep the skin and arteries supple and the body warm.

Essential fatty acids are especially important if you have PMS and if you suffer from any of the following, all of which can be signs of EFA deficiency: dry skin, hair loss, lifeless hair, poor wound-healing, dandruff, depression, irritability, soft or brittle nails, dry eyes, fatigue, aching joints, weight gain, high blood pressure and arthritis.

Aren't we always told that cutting down on fat is good for us? That's exactly what I did. I cut down drastically, but I now realize that I cut down too drastically. You need to include some fat in your diet, but it has to be the right kind. I had no idea that my low moods, my dry hair and weight gain were related to the lack of essential fats in my diet. Within weeks of taking fish oil supplements not only did I feel more energetic and less moody, but my PMS got better and I started to see the scales go down instead of up. **Sarah, 30**

This week we would like to focus on perhaps the most crucial essential fatty acid if you have PMS: Omega-3. You need to include Omega-3 in your PMS eating plan because it can decrease inflammation, help stabilize blood sugar, fight acne and increase the production of feel-good hormones.

You can find Omega-3 in the fat or oil of coldwater fish such as herring, salmon, tuna and sardines. Fish oil is also a good source of vitamin D, which helps the body absorb those essential PMS-beating minerals: calcium and magnesium.

To ensure that you include enough Omega-3 fatty acid in your diet, eat two to five coldwater fish meals per week. Other good sources include fish oil, flaxseed oil, walnuts, nuts and soybeans. You'll notice that we've included lots of these ingredients in tomorrow's meal plan to get you thinking along the right lines.

As a rule of thumb, if you eat plenty of fish, take fish oil or take flaxseed oil, you should be getting enough Omega-3.

EXERCISE

Give yourself a day off from your walk today (and remember on the day when you do your exercise class you don't need to do your walk either), but do make sure that you do your stretching and that you are as active as possible during the day. If your job involves a lot of sitting, make sure that every 30 minutes or so you get up and stretch, jog on the spot or go for a short walk around the room.

EMOTIONAL WELL-BEING

Have there been times when you just lost it over something really trivial? Let us reassure you that, however weird or crazy you get when you are premenstrual, you are not alone. This kind of angry outburst isn't unusual. Millions of women with PMS have moments when they feel out of control, confused, tense or angry with themselves.

> *I had some errands to run, so I asked my family to tidy the kitchen before I get back. When I get back it is exactly as I left it and everyone is watching television. Something inside me explodes. For a moment I am crazy with anger. I scream at my family. The kids start crying, my partner looks shocked. I run outside slamming the door and take off in my car. I drive around the block, still fuming. When I come back my family is tidying the kitchen. Nobody speaks as I walk in. I go to the bedroom and start crying. I think I'm a horrible mother and a horrible wife.* **Penny, 31**

> *Mood swings are ruining my life. I thought mood swings were all about highs and lows, but for me the highs are rare. Two weeks out of four I feel OK. Not great, just OK. The rest of the time I'll be doing things I normally do and then suddenly burst into tears over nothing. With no warning I just snap. I sometimes think I must be going mad.* **Jo, 29**

Many women with PMS talk about feeling separated from themselves or feeling out of control or not knowing who they really are. Each month there are emotional extremes with angry blow-ups at one end of the spectrum and guilt and despair at the other. You have an angry outburst and feel guilty about it afterwards. You promise not to let yourself get so out of control again. You can't believe what you did. You decide that this wasn't you.

Then for reasons you can't understand, you become angry and it happens again. Only now things are worse because you have let yourself down. You didn't keep a promise to yourself. You feel like a worthless person. This is when guilt kicks in.

The guilt starts when you start to blame yourself for not being able to control your behaviour. This inability to control the situation – the anger and the guilt – can be the most devastating part of suffering from PMS, often more upsetting than the physical symptoms.

Knowledge and willpower alone cannot overcome your problem – however many positive-thinking books you read. What will make the difference is what you are doing right now – changing your lifestyle one step at a time. That's why this week we are going to look at ways you can combat the feelings of anger, tension, anxiety, frustration, irritability, guilt and confusion that can come up with PMS.

The first step we'd like you to take today is simple. All we want you to do is re-read the information above again and remind yourself that mood swings or a flash of anger or tension in the week or so before your period can be caused by hormonal fluctuations.

We'd like you to go easy on yourself and stop tearing yourself down. We'd like you to understand, really understand, that PMS affects not just your body but your mood as well.

Try to get the idea into your head that you are suffering from a medical problem – one that will improve with the changes you are making. Establish for yourself that you may act out of control during the week or so before your period, but that you can deal calmly and rationally with the same issues when you are not premenstrual. Give yourself permission to forgive yourself for events in the past so you can move forward to more positive things.

Day 2

NUTRITION

Sample Menu
Breakfast and supplements: Scrambled free-range egg on wholemeal toast with scraping of butter, glass of organic diluted apple juice or calcium-enriched soymilk

Snack: Sesame seed bar, glass of calcium-enriched soy or nut milk or organic skimmed or semi-skimmed milk
Lunch: Fish and potato pie, green salad with mint, tomato and basil; slice of fruit loaf*
Snack: Fresh fruit salad sprinkled with cottage cheese and nuts
Dinner: Lentil soup*, lean meat, fish or tofu with pilau rice and vegetable stir fry; brulee*

Task for Today

Yesterday we looked at increasing the amount of Omega-3 essential fatty acid in your diet. We'd like you to continue thinking about this today and for the rest of the plan. If you think you aren't eating enough, it might be a good idea to take fatty acids in supplement form, in addition to your multivitamin and -mineral and your extra calcium and magnesium supplements. Try 1 teaspoonful or 1,000 mg in capsule form daily of flaxseed oil, or a high-strength Omega-3 fish oil capsule.

EXERCISE

Do your 30-minute walk and stretching routine today. Also give your local leisure centre a call or visit and check out the times and prices to go swimming. After walking, swimming is one of the safest and most effective ways to exercise. It's also great fun. Plan to go sometime this week and, when you do go, limit the amount of time you sit and splash – swim as much as you can. If you work you might be able to pop in some time this week during your lunch hour or before you travel home. It's a great way to unwind.

EMOTIONAL WELL-BEING

Promise yourself today that the next time you lose it you won't punish yourself. Give yourself a break. Today be kind, patient and generous with yourself. Do something that you enjoy, like browsing in a bookstore or going for a walk or taking a long, hot bath. Think about the things you do to help other people, and try doing a few for yourself today.

Think about asking for the support of those around you and not withdrawing if you engage in another angry outburst. Call or talk to your loved ones. Alienating yourself from others is not the answer. You need the understanding and support of family and friends. If you live alone, go somewhere where you won't feel completely alone, like a swimming pool or shopping mall. Just hang around with other people. Withdrawing from others makes the situation worse, not better. Let other people know what is going on so that they can support you through it.

Day 3

NUTRITION

Sample Menu
Breakfast and supplements: Oatmeal made with skimmed milk, low-fat yogurt, glass of fresh-pressed apple juice
Snack: 2 digestive biscuits with cottage cheese, glass of calcium-enriched skimmed milk
Lunch: Vegetable soup*, 2 slices of wholemeal toast; fresh fruit salad with sprinkling of seeds and raisins
Snack: Small flapjack
Dinner: Jacket potato with lean meat, fish or tofu, baked beans, fruity carrot salad*; banana surprise*

Task for Today
Remember if it is the right kind of fat, fat can be very good for you. Too much of the wrong kind of fat can trigger symptoms or make them worse. So this week make sure you watch your intake of saturated fat, which is found in red meat, bacon, cheese, full-fat dairy produce and tropical oils like palm and coconut. Saturated fats can contribute to weight gain, block other nutrients from doing their job effectively, trigger the production of bad prostaglandins and interfere with the body's absorption of fatty acids that you need to beat PMS.

This also holds true for hydrogenated fats, which are found in margarine, fast foods, crisps, biscuits and crackers and rancid vegetable oils. The process of hydrogenation, which makes a fat more spreadable, changes the essential fatty acids into transfatty acids. These not only upset hormonal balance but have been linked to all sorts of health problems, including heart disease. So skip the cheeseburger with fries and go for some delicious baked fish with lemon and olive oil instead. Skip the margarine and use butter or unhydrogenated margarine instead.

Monounsaturated fats are not classed as essential fatty acids but they can boost your health. Olive oil is high in monosaturated fats which are thought to lower the risk of heart disease. Wherever possible buy organic cold-pressed unrefined vegetables oils or extra virgin olive oil, because they are less likely to have nutrients and chemicals extracted during manufacturing. Cooking oils can be easily damaged, so you need to take care when storing and using them. If oils are overheated, left to stand too long in sunlight or reused after cooking, they lose their benefits. If you use cold-pressed vegetable oil, keep it sealed in the fridge, away from heat, light and air, and only use cold in salad dressing or instead of butter on your jacket potato or peas.

Here's a reference table for you to use. Why not stick it on your fridge?

FATS THAT HARM		
Bacon bits	Butter	Cream
Cream cheese	Lard	Sour cream
Vegetable shortening	Refined oils	Pork
High-fat dairy produce	Roasted seeds and nuts	Beef
Lamb	Eggs	Coconut
FATS THAT HEAL		
Evening primrose oil	Cold-pressed vegetable oil	Avocados
Almonds	Sesame seeds	Sunflower seeds
Chicken	Seaweed	Walnuts
Soybeans	Linseed (Flaxseed)	Hemp
Olive oil	Olives	

EXERCISE

Do your 30-minute walk and your stretching. If swimming isn't your cup of tea, find out about dance classes in your area. We recommend jive dancing. It's great exercise and, whether you go with or without a partner, you'll find it's terrific fun. You could also try belly dancing – excellent for toning the pelvic region, boosting body image and toning the waist. Or how about salsa for co-ordination or a romantic night out? You can choose so many forms of dance, from ballet or tap to ballroom or disco to line dancing, that it's really worth exploring the options to make exercise fun.

EMOTIONAL WELL-BEING

Managing anger is something all of us need to work on, not just those who have PMS.

Anger is not a 'bad' emotion. In fact, anger can be very helpful. Feeling angry can be a great motivator to accomplish important things. For example, anger at injustice rights many wrongs in the world.

Refusing to acknowledge we are angry and turning our anger inward can cause depression. A recent study shows that this is implicated in heart disease, too. But letting ourselves explode with anger is unhealthy as well. In *The Dance of Anger: A Woman's Guide to Changing the Patterns of Intimate Relationships*, Harriet Goldhor Lerner says that venting our anger does no good unless we also change the unhealthy ways we relate to others. She identifies two common patterns in women: the nice lady and the bitch.

Nice ladies are afraid to express anger even when expressing their feelings is justified. These women tend to explode at inappropriate times and end up feeling guilty.

Bitchy women spend too much energy trying to change other people instead of focusing on themselves.

Both ways of relating make women feel powerless and lead to further anger.

If you lose it by having a temper-tantrum or going into a rage, what is in control? Your anger is – you are not. So your task for today is to consider one word, which The Institute of Mental Health suggests when you get angry: RETHINK.

- R stands for **Recognize**. Recognize and acknowledge your anger. Remind yourself that feeling anger isn't bad. Anger can be very useful. The important thing is how you channel that anger.
- E stands for **Empathize**. The dictionary defines empathy as 'understanding so intimate that the feelings, thought and motives of one are readily comprehended by another'. In other words, try to understand where another person is coming from. This can be hard when you are feeling mad, but give it a try. Perhaps the person who cut in front of you in traffic has had a bad day, too, or simply didn't see you.
- T is for **Think**. Try thinking about the anger-inducing incident in a new and different way. Perhaps you can see some humour in the situation? Did you have a part to play in the problem? Do you have any ideas for solving it?
- H is for **Hear**. Really listen to what the other person has to say/their point of view. Repeat back what you think you have heard.
- I is for **Integrate**. Integrate love and respect in your response. Use 'I' messages to state your opinion on how what happened made you feel. 'I' messages are statements about how you feel as opposed to statements condemning another person's behaviour. For example 'I get upset when I am interrupted,' not 'You never listen.'
- N stands for **Notice**. Take note of what works in controlling your anger: exercise, writing down your feelings in your emotional diary, hot baths, hugs?
- K stands for **Keep** your focus on the present. Don't drag up old grudges.

Now let's see this working in action. Say someone at work has taken your favourite mug and used up all your milk. You've had a terrible journey to work and are gasping for a cuppa. You know who has taken it and you want to strangle her. She never brings her own things. Trouble is, she is in a meeting right now. You'd like to give her a piece of your mind. But wait.

You've written RETHINK on the back of your hand. Let's try this new method:

- Recognize your anger. No problems there.
- Empathize? See her viewpoint. Well, you have borrowed things from her in the past, too.
- Think about the situation in a new way. Her birthday is next week; perhaps you could buy her a new mug.
- Listen to her. She isn't here now but listen to what she has to say. Perhaps she will apologize.
- Integrate love and respect. Mug-pinching aside, you do like and respect this woman.
- Notice what works in controlling your anger. It helps you to write things down. Perhaps you could write her a note.
- Keep your attention in the present. You have to. Your day is too busy to think about who borrows whose mug at work.

If RETHINK is too hard to remember, visualize a traffic light: red, yellow and green.

- **Red**: Stop. Don't react. Take a few moments to reflect.
- **Yellow**: Take your time – maybe until the end of your PMS phase.
- **Green**: Find the person with whom you have disagreed. Talk things over.

Day 4

NUTRITION

Sample Menu
Breakfast with supplements: Porridge oats with skimmed milk, dried apricots and sultanas, glass of fresh-pressed orange juice
Snack: Apple with handful of nuts
Lunch: Dahl* with wholegrain rice; fruit salad and low-fat yogurt
Snack: Slice of plum bread with glass of calcium-enriched skimmed milk
Dinner: Lean meat or fish, medium jacket potato, large helping of vegetables or salad; baked apples with low-fat ice cream

Task for Today

Today, make a point of checking out your local health food shop. If you have never been before and it all looks very daunting, don't worry, it's really just like going to your local supermarket or chemist. You will find a range of healthy food choices and supplements along with a variety of herbal or alternative remedies for common ailments. You may also find that the shop has lots of information (leaflets or books) for you to browse through, or even a computer database packed with fascinating information about ways to boost your health and well-being. It's a great place to visit and we hope that you will become a regular there over the weeks ahead.

For today we'd like you to explore all the options for oils, foods and supplements rich in essential fatty acids, such as hemp oil, seeds and nuts, and evening primrose oil. Ask for help if you need to. Have a think and then decide which foods, oils and/or supplements you are going to include in your diet on a daily basis to boost your health and well-being over the weeks ahead.

EXERCISE

Do your 30-minute walk and your stretching. We'd also like you to start doing some sit-ups.

Just before you go to bed – or better still, as soon as you get up in the morning, do some abdominal curls. We recommend that you start with 10 and build up over the weeks to about 50.

> Lie flat on your back on the floor, bending your knees to reduce the strain on your lower back.
> From here, supporting your head with both hands, curl forwards gently to lift your upper back off the ground, breathing out as you do.
> Slowly lower yourself down, breathing in.
> If possible don't let your head touch the ground between sit-ups, but if you aren't there yet, don't worry. Do what you can.

EMOTIONAL WELL-BEING
Try this if you feel tension rising today, or jot it down for future use. It's a great technique to have on stand-by:

1. Call a mental time out
Instead of taking charge right now, try letting go of tension. Take a moment to tell yourself. 'Wait a minute. Right now I can't handle this. I need to take a breather.'

2. Take a breather – literally
Take a deep breath. Let it in slowly through your mouth, filling your chest, feeling your diaphragm expand – and let it out quickly through your mouth. Hear yourself make a quiet huffing noise like you would if you were using your breath to clean a pair of sunglasses.

3. Puff the anger and tension out
Take another deep breath … in and out … rolling your shoulders to stretch and release any tension you have gathered there. Repeat, letting your ribs expand and focusing on releasing tension there. Again, let the intake of air cause your diaphragm and lower abdomen to fill the way a baby's tummy rises when she breathes – and focus on releasing stress caught in your mid-section.

4. See the anger go … Hear peace return
Just refocusing your mind from the external pressures and onto your breathing may be enough to calm you. An additional step may help:
In your mind's eye, picture your anger as an object – a feather or a mist – that you are blowing away from you each time you exhale. As you let the anger go, repeat a positive affirmation like 'I am calm.' Listen for that small, still voice to speak calming words to you.

Day 5

NUTRITION

Sample Menu

Breakfast with supplements: Half a grapefruit sprinkled with nuts and seeds, 2 slices of wholemeal bread with scraping of butter and honey, glass of calcium-enriched skimmed milk
Snack: Low-fat yogurt sprinkled with almonds
Lunch: Vegetable soup*, large salad with nut oil dressing and sesame seeds; fresh fruit
Snack: Smoothie* that includes a splash of hemp seed oil
Dinner: Potato omelette* with vegetables; fruit crumble with chopped almonds

Task for Today

Today we'd like to think again about creative ways you can include nuts, seeds and essential fatty acids with each meal: nuts and seeds sprinkled onto your food or added during the cooking process to add extra flavour, green leafy salads sprinkled with nut oil dressing, lean meat cooked with olive oil, a smoothie that includes a dash of hemp seed oil. There are so many great ways you can include essential fatty acids in your diet. Not only do essential fatty acids make your meals more tasty and satisfying, they boost your health and help you beat PMS, too.

EXERCISE
Do your 30-minute walk, your stretching and your sit-ups.

EMOTIONAL WELL-BEING
Remember, having PMS and feeling emotional can go hand in hand. Today, think about your moods as one current pouring into the river of your running thoughts. Sitting or walking by yourself focuses on the emotions going on inside you. Watching how your emotions can change and colour your thoughts is like watching food colouring swirl in a cake batter. You can see how they affect you. So:

- Observe how you are feeling ('I've been tense all morning').
- Observe the topics you are thinking about (job, home, friends). When we are in balance our thoughts tend to be balanced and neutral, not negative.
- Observe how your mood is pulling your thoughts into the current.
- Observe how turning up the flow of reason soothes the mood flow. See tips on doing this in our positive thinking section (pages 111–12). Talking logically to the negative thoughts created by your emotions will turn down the mental stress they cause.

If you use this strategy you can take charge of emotionally charged thoughts. It will stop you feeling like you are losing it or going crazy during difficult times in your cycle.

But what if you just haven't the energy to do much about the emotions charging around in your head? When you feel so tense that you feel overwhelmed, try this technique:

1 If possible, step outside of your immediate circumstances. Excuse yourself from a meeting, take a break from the kids, pull the car over. Changing your setting adds to the sense of leaving mental stress behind. If you can't leave the location, try this:

2 Focus your eyes intently on a fixed spot about 2 or 3 feet ahead of you.
When you are tense, every part of you tends to bear down. Muscles tense. Notice that you are most likely looking down. Now feel that tension in your body, face, forehead and eyes.

3 Let your eyes drift upwards. Let your focus broaden until you are staring into the distance.

Refocusing your gaze can help you reverse feelings of tension and anxiety. Letting your eyes drift up – until they reach the sky or a spot on the wall – triggers a relaxation response that spreads from your head to your whole body. You will probably find that you also take a deep breathe as you do this. Keep breathing deeply and feel how the release of muscle tension re-establishes mental calm.

By letting these quick strategies do their work you can re-enter the room you stepped away from and not allow PMS to rob you of that 'in charge' feeling you need.

Day 6

NUTRITION

Sample Menu
Breakfast with supplements: Poached egg on wholemeal toast, low-fat yogurt sprinked with nuts, glass of fresh-pressed apple juice
Snack: Smoothie with sesame seed crackers
Lunch: Vegetable mixed grill with tomatoes, courgettes and aubergine, marinade made with sunflower oil, lemon juice, tomato puree, chilli powder, paprika and thyme; fresh fruit salad with chopped almonds
Snack: Small flapjack, glass of skimmed milk
Dinner: Lasagna with beans*; baked apple with honey and raisins

Task for Today
Please re-read all the information on phytoestrogens (page 22), magnesium (pages 270–1), calcium (page 269) and the information on essential fatty acids that we've discussed this week. Now explore your recipe books (buy a recipe book if you don't have one or take one out from the library) and start planning menus for tomorrow and for the week ahead. If you are going shopping today or tomorrow, make sure you write out a list of the ingredients you will need before you get to the supermarket.

EXERCISE
Do your 30-minute walk, your stretching and your sit-ups.

EMOTIONAL WELL-BEING
At your own pace, re-read the information and have a go at some of the exercises from Days 1 to 5 this week. Write down how you feel before and after in your emotions diary.

It's good to take time out to explore your emotions. Keeping feelings stifled for too long is bad for your health and will certainly make PMS mood swings worse. Better to find a way to express your feelings and let them go. You don't want to go round yelling at people, but you can find other ways to express yourself! Your emotions diary can help you here.

Sometimes, too, it is better to take the risk and express your feelings in a direct and assertive way instead of bottling up your anger. Learn to initiate frank dialogues with people who make you feel tense and angry. Talk it out. Be courteous but direct. When you are feeling bad, say so, both to yourself and to others. The same holds true when you are alone. If you feel like crying, moaning, punching a pillow, shouting out loud or yelling in the shower, go ahead and let fly. It's OK to feel hurt. It's OK to feel anger. There is nothing improper or crazy about these activities, and in many cases the sense of release they generate helps clear your psychological air.

Day 7

NUTRITION
Have fun today planning, cooking and eating your own PMS-friendly meals. Take your supplements with breakfast, use our sample recipes from the last four weeks to guide you, and don't forget you can always refer to the recipes in Appendix 3.

EXERCISE
Do your 30-minute walk, stretching and sit-ups. We'd also like you to start paying more attention to your posture over the weeks ahead. Holding your body in the correct position is one of the most important factors in maintaining good health. Our skeletons are designed to hold the weight of our body as close to the centre of gravity as possible. The further our skeleton is pulled away from this natural alignment (tummy sticking out, shoulders slumped and so on), the higher the incidence of muscle and joint problems. In addition to this your posture also sends subconscious signals to other people. Those who are able to maintain good posture are

perceived as more attractive than those who cannot. Changing your posture will change the way you look at the world as well as the way the world looks at you.

Here are some things for you to think about this weekend:

Good posture is critical to well-being. Too much slumping as we walk, sit or eat will potentially put undue pressure on the spine and aging back trouble and joint pain are virtually inevitable. But what is good posture?

Good posture has nothing to do with the old school rigidity of pulling in your stomach and puffing your chest out. Good posture is about looking effortlessly pulled up. It is about ease of movement and freedom and using the minimum amount of effort to keep the body upright.

Life can be stressful and it can be hard to obtain this ideal. We are needlessly tensing and straining our bodies all day long and waste energy. We don't observe proper body mechanics and pull the whole out of line. Small wonder that we get 'unexplained' aches and pains, sleepless night and mood swings. All too often improper body mechanics – and not PMS – are causing the tension.

When we start to become aware of the degree of tension in our bodies we can start to make positive changes. Once we stop all the distortions, we may well find that aches and pains disappear, and that we are a little taller, have more energy and feel better.

When muscles become less tense we return energy to our bodies, according to East Asian traditions of medicine who call this energy Qi. Qi travels through the body along pathways, and when Qi gets blocked, this is when ill-health occurs. Energy and well-being can be restored by getting the energy flowing again – and we can do this by releasing the tension we store away in our muscles.

Proprioception is the term used for the process that keeps the body in a state of alignment. Muscle spindles alongside the muscle fibres supply the brain with a continual flow of information via the spinal cord and nerves, and in turn receive the instructions to keep us in balance. There are various techniques which can help us tune in to this inner balance: yoga, t'ai chi, martial arts and Alexander Technique, for example.

Realignment methods may have different philosophies behind them but the goal is often the same: a free, supple, lengthened body that resists the tendency we have to contract, which causes many of the discomforts we wrongly associate with getting older.

Common to all these methods is the emphasis on doing the minimum so that only the relevant muscles are brought into play. As physical effort diminishes, mental clarity and inner harmony increase. We understand our bodies from the inside out rather than the outside in. We begin to appreciate just how remarkable our body is and are less self-critical as we concentrate on whole-body awareness.

If you don't want to take up a realignment method to improve your posture, there are ways you can work on your posture yourself. First of all, you need to become aware that the muscles of alignment are situated at the back of your body, not the front. That is why sucking in your tummy or pulling back your shoulders often don't improve your shape. The muscles at the front of the body are not meant to be stabilizing, but the muscles that run along the back and spine and legs are. As we are not used to using these muscles at first, they may need retraining. This may explain why you may find it hard to stand balanced on both feet rather than shifting from one to the other, or to sit with your legs uncrossed.

Fortunately, once you start thinking of the back-to-front way, muscles don't take long to get back into operation and it won't seem so tiring. Once you get used to lengthening, your stomach naturally flattens and your shape improves.

To do a quick check on your posture have a look at yourself sideways in a mirror. Try to tuck your bottom under and pull upward. Lift your head and chin up and feel as if someone is pulling you from the centre of your head with a string. If you compare how you look now you will realize how slumped you normally are. You'll also see how good posture can take pounds off you and make you look more confident and poised.

Alongside posture, proper body mechanics are also important to avoid strain and tension. When bending or lifting, plant your feet firmly apart and bend your knees so that your back stays long. Hold an object you are lifting close to you and lift it by straightening your knees, not your back. Pull up when you sit, too, and try to avoid crossing your legs. This can be a hard habit to break, but if you continue it will really weaken your lower back muscles.

Work at desks that are the right height for you and that help you keep your back long. When driving, make sure your knees are slightly higher than your hips. And if you must wear high heels, wear them for short periods only. High heels shift the centre of gravity forward, distort your posture and put your body under tremendous strain.

EMOTIONAL WELL-BEING

Dr Dean Ornish, a leading spokesman for the natural approach to a healthy heart, believes that deep breathing is one of the simplest yet most effective stress- and anger-management techniques there is. At the Preventative Medicine Research Institute in Sausalito, California, Ornish and his team have developed several highly effective stress-management programmes that centre on breathing therapy, many of which are derived from the age-old principles of yoga.

You don't have to enrol in a health-care institute to put deep breathing exercises to work. Today we'd like you to practise some of the following techniques at home or at work, to use whenever you feel tense or angry. You'll be pleased to see how much deep breathing can calm you down even in the most volatile of situations. Try the following:

- When you have a quiet moment, sit up in a chair and practise a few minutes of deep breathing. Breathe in on a count of seven, hold for a count of three, then exhale for a count of seven. Do ten repetitions. Do this exercise first thing in the morning, last thing at night, mid-morning, lunchtime and teatime. The good effects will influence your whole day.

- If you feel agitated, stop what you are doing and take several deep breaths. Wait a few moments and then repeat. This little trick can really help you get back on track in times of chaos and confusion.

When practising deep breathing, remember what we've said earlier about 'tummy breathing'. Breathe first into your stomach, then into your mid-section and then into your lower and upper chest in one single flowing motion. Breathing in this way ensures that your chest cavity is filled with air, your lungs are properly exercised and oxygen intake is maximized. At various times in the day, make a conscious effort to breathe more deeply from your stomach to bring more oxygen into your system. This will make a noticeable difference in your overall stress level. Programme yourself to take these deep breaths whenever you feel tense. For example, take a few breaths before answering the phone or walking into a room full of strangers.

Don't forget the importance of the out-breath when you do your deep breathing. We often tend to concentrate on inhaling, forgetting that vigorous exhalation rids the lungs of stale air and removes toxins. For maximum relaxation, deep inhalation and deep exhalation are of equal importance.

VITALITY BOOSTER

Having More Fun

This week, think about ways to have more fun. It may be hard for you to find time for pleasure in your life, but it is essential. Regularly having fun is one of the five central factors in leading a satisfied life. Studies[1] have shown that people who spend time enjoying themselves are more likely to feel happy on a daily basis and more likely to feel comfortable with their age and stage in life.

Pleasure plays an important role in everyday life, but it is undervalued and under-explored in both science and society, according to ARISE (Associates for Research Into the Science of Enjoyment), an organization that was established in order to create a better understanding of the benefits of pleasure. ARISE encourages research into the subject and provides a forum for the presentation and discussion of the various aspects of enjoyment. It believes that pleasurable activities, enjoyed in moderation, make a positive contribution to and are part of a balanced and well-rounded approach to life.

Pleasure is important to health in two ways. First, it can act proactively to promote good physical and mental health and protect against ill-health (inoculation). Secondly, it can aid the process of unwinding and protect against recent unpleasant experiences (antidote). Research shows that experiencing pleasure leads to a reduction in the stress hormones such as cortisol, and strengthens the immune response – therefore offering us greater resistance to infections and disease.

It's official – having fun is essential in your life and good for your health and well-being. So this week, take some time to plan for pleasure.

There's a whole range of leisure pursuits you can choose from. Some may be quite demanding like playing football or squash; others may be gentle and relaxing like a game of golf, but they are all sources of pleasure and a chance to improve your skills. You may want to take up a hobby. Hobbies are a steady source of pleasure, providing two essential ingredients: consistency and fun. In surveys[2] of thousands of adults, those who had a hobby were found to be more likely to feel happy with themselves and their lives. Other studies[3] show that hobbies or leisure that involve other people provide social support that can help us manage stress. One study showed that people with fewer community ties were more likely to fall ill than those who had strong ties. Your hobby could be anything from painting to pottery, learning a new language to knitting, organizing a book group, going to the cinema or even walking in the country.

If you know what makes you feel great, then go ahead and clear time in your diary this week and over the weeks ahead for it. If you aren't so sure, you may need to do a little detective work. Think about your emotions and happiness. What makes your heart sing?

Think money is the answer? Why do so many instant millionaires report that their money brings them more misery than joy? A study of life satisfaction[4] looked at 20 different factors that might contribute to happiness. Nineteen of these factors did matter, and one did not. The one factor that did not matter was financial status. Prosperity is not always related to how much money you have in the bank. Why are some people with less money happier than others? Studies[5] show that what people like most about their lives isn't money or status, but feeling fulfilled and interested. Ask any young lover, first-time mother or Olympic athlete.

You might want to take an evening class in something that has always interested you. The Internet is a great place for information-gathering. If something fascinates you, write a letter to an expert, initiate a meeting with them, buy a diary and start writing down all the things that you think will make you happy. Write down what you are best at, and what other people compliment you on most, such as how organized you are or how you are such a laugh. After a day or so, reread that diary. Think about the best moments in your life, the best holidays in your life. Do these have anything in common?

Plan dinner parties and invite people you don't know very well. Ask them questions about their lives, what they enjoy and what they want to do next. For one day, or one week even, avoid talking about yourself and ask people lots of questions about them.

One way to find out what you enjoy is to try something that seems unusual, offbeat, adventurous or even silly. Plan an afternoon in which you do something you have never tried before, just because it sounds interesting – like going to a dance class, having a full-body massage, going to a new pub with friends, visiting a funfair with your kids and going on the rides with them, even walking barefoot on the sand. Do some volunteer work, take up an unusual hobby or part-time job. Draw up a business plan for something that just sounds like fun. Then think about what you liked and disliked about this new experience, and how it surprised you. You never know what you might discover about yourself.

The point of these exercises is to make you step back from your life and really start to see if there are connections among the things you enjoy or feel energized by. When you listen to other people or try out new things, what really makes you feel excited? What is fun for you? If you are studying, reading, looking, listening, gathering information and considering your options and you still aren't sure what makes your heart sing, you could try looking into your past. Was there once something that made you happy, like horse-riding or singing, but got left behind because you thought you had outgrown it? Think about those dreams which you have always longed for but have had to put aside because other things got in the way. Are you ready to go for them now?

Don't beat yourself up if you find that your interests and your passions change as you get older. Sometimes we just outgrow interests or passions and need to find new ones to motivate and energize us all over again. The important thing isn't so much what you are doing but the spirit in which you are doing it. Are you having fun on a regular basis? Make sure this week and every week from now on that, alongside your responsibilities, you also schedule in time for pleasure even if this involves a regular trip away, days or evenings out, or something as simple as an hour in your bath with a book that makes you laugh.

And finally, if some of your enjoyment centres around things like alcohol, chocolate, caffeine, gambling or bungy jumpy which aren't 100 per cent good for you, remember the 80/20 rule that we established at the beginning of the book. You can extend this rule to your lifestyle, too. As long as you do things which are good for you *most* of the time, you can allow yourself the occasional treat or adrenaline rush now and again!

Week 5

Day 1

NUTRITION

There are no sample menus today because from now on we would like you to create your own menus for the rest of the plan. You can, of course, go back to Week 1 and repeat all the menus from Weeks 1 to 4 for Weeks 5 to 8. Whatever you decide, enjoy your food and don't forget to take your multivitamin and -mineral supplement and your calcium and magnesium supplement every morning. Also try to use some of the PMS-friendly recipes in Appendix 3 for guidance.

EXERCISE

Muscle-building is equally important as aerobic exercise. Strong, toned muscles help maintain your metabolism. Even when you are relaxing, your muscles are burning calories. Fat, on the other hand, just sits there and burns no calories. Scientists have worked out that people who strength-train can improve their metabolic rate by 15 per cent. This can make a huge difference to achieving your weight-management goals, if you have them.

All this week, along with your daily 30-minute aerobic workout, we are going to suggest simple toning exercises you can do at home.

In order to strengthen your muscles and make them look lean and firm you need to use resistance. The best way is to use your body weight and challenge as many muscle groups as you can. The type of exercises we are recommending this week are a bit like a circuit, meaning that you repeat the exercises and then have a rest between each set. Start slowly and work to the point of mild exertion. You should do about 10 to 15 repetitions for each exercise, at first counting to 2 on the upward phase and 2 on the downward phase. You should breathe out when you exert effort. This week we would like you to start with one set (10 repetitions) of each exercise.

Push-ups
Lie flat on the floor with your hands shoulder-width apart, upper arms parallel to the ground. Push up on your toes, keeping your body straight until your elbows extend. Just before your elbows lock, slowly lower and repeat. You might like to start on your knees if it is a bit too hard to do this on your toes.

Upper body stretch
When you have done 10 to 15 push-ups, do an upper-body stretch. Stand up and imagine you are holding a big beach ball with your arms. Hold this position for 30 seconds.

Don't forget to do your 30-minute walk today, too.

EMOTIONAL WELL-BEING
Today we are going to look at your emotional relationship with food. There is a reason why certain foods can brighten your mood and others can lower it. Within your brain, chemicals help transmit messages from one nerve cell to another. Two of these chemicals – serotonin and norepinephrine – affect the way you feel. Your body makes these endorphins from the food you eat – so you can, to some extent, influence your mood by eating certain foods.

Not surprisingly, the main source of endorphins are sugary, carbohydrate-rich foods. This is why biscuits, chocolate, white bread and white rice appear to be so comforting. But as you know the problem with eating these foods is that as sugar enters your bloodstream too quickly, along with a rush of serotonin you get a rush of insulin, something women with PMS need to avoid. Blood sugar and endorphin levels both drop, and you feel hungry again and worse than you did before.

Write down in your diary how hungry you are before eating, and how you feel physically, mentally and emotionally. Then write down what you eat and drink, and how you feel physically, mentally and emotionally after eating.

Becoming more aware of your feelings when you eat will help you to become more attuned to hunger signals. We all, at times, pop things into our mouths without thinking about it. The problem is that if you are not concentrating on your food you don't notice when you are full, and by the time you do you may have overindulged. So today and for the rest of this week, the next time you want to eat, get into the habit of asking yourself if you are really hungry. If you aren't sure, you probably aren't. Ask yourself if anything other than food – like a walk, a chat or a hug – would satisfy you instead.

Day 2

NUTRITION
Today we'd like you to re-read the information about sugar cravings in Week 3 (page 113) and why eating too much sugar isn't a good idea if you have PMS.

On average, Western women eat about 90 g/3¼ oz of sugar a day. In an ideal PMS-free diet, you would eat only two servings (30g) a day.

> **What Is a Serving of Sugar or Sugary Foods?**
> 15 g or 1tbsp of sugar
> 1 rounded tsp jam/honey
> 2 biscuits
> half a slice of cake or a doughnut or danish pastry
> 1 small bar of chocolate
> 1 small tube or bag of sweets

If you eat more sugary food than this, you should try to make small changes over the weeks ahead. Here are some useful tips:

- Limit your intake of sugar and added sugar to two servings a day.
- Start to cut down on sugar in drinks and on breakfast cereals. Sweeten cereals with fruit instead.
- Avoid white and refined foods.
- Keep fresh fruit, dried fruit and healthy snacks nearby so you won't be tempted to reach for a chocolate bar.
- Eat whole foods – whole grains, nuts seeds, fresh fruit and vegetables.
- Dilute fruit juices and only eat dried fruit in small quantities.
- If you do get a craving for sweet food eat fruit instead of sweet snacks, or other sweet foods, such as malt loaf, which at least include nourishment along with their sugar rush. Get some hot chocolate and drink some with soy or skimmed milk.
- Explore your health food shop for healthy snacking options. For example, rice cakes with peanut butter make a great snack.
- Smelling vanilla essence oil can help prevent cravings for sweet food, according to research from St George's Medical Hospital, London. Dab a couple of drops on a tissue and inhale when you feel the need.

EXERCISE
Do your 30-minute walk, your push-ups and add some squats (see page 166). Finish with your stretching routine.

> **Squats**
> With your feet shoulder-width apart and facing forward, slowly
> bend at the knees and lower your body until your thighs are
> parallel to the floor. Look straight ahead and keep your back as
> straight as you can, then slowly stand up again. Repeat this
> exercise 10 times.

EMOTIONAL WELL-BEING

Pete Cohen and Judith Verity from Lighten Up Weight Loss Consultancy in
the UK believe that there is no such thing as an unhealthy food, only an
unhealthy attitude towards food. If you can change your attitude you can
eat healthily without feeling stressed or depressed, and you can deal with
your emotions in a more positive way. Instead of banning foods, which
will only make you obsess about them, think about this today: *Food is not
your enemy.* Write this down and pin it to your fridge door.

Focus your thoughts today on how PMS symptoms will improve through
healthier eating habits. The next time you are tempted to eat something
which you know is going to lead to weight-gain and a worsening of your
symptoms, ask yourself if you really enjoy it. Wouldn't it be better to
choose the healthier alternative?

Day 3

NUTRITION

How Much Food Are You Really Eating?
The easiest way to reduce your food intake without losing out on valuable
nutrients is to cut down on your portion size. As a rough guide, according
to the US Department of Agriculture you need:

- 2 to 3 servings of dairy products (milk, yogurt, cheese) or calcium-
  enriched non-dairy products like soy or nut milk a day. One serving is
  about 2 oz of cheese or 1 cup of milk or yogurt.

- 2 to 3 servings of meat, fish, eggs, beans and nuts a day. One serving is 1 egg or half a cup of beans, or meat or fish about the size of a pack of playing cards.
- 5 to 6 servings of whole grains a day. One serving is 1 slice of bread, a bowl of cereal or half a cup of rice or pasta.
- 4 servings of fruit. One serving is one piece of fruit.
- 5 or more servings of vegetables. One servings is half a cup of cooked vegetables, 1 cup of raw
- Fats and oils to be eaten sparingly.

If you have weight to lose, start checking your serving size and make a few small reductions. You don't need to cut out all the foods you enjoy, you just need to eat less of them.

EXERCISE
Do your 30-minute walk, your push-ups, squats and add some oblique sits-ups (see below). Finish with your stretching routine.

> **Oblique Sit-ups**
> Lie flat on the floor, bend your knees and place your arms in the air. From this position roll onto your left hip and shoulder so that your knees point away from you to the right. Use your left arm to support your neck and keep your right arm on the floor. Then slowly reach your left elbow towards your left hip, rotating your body and crunching up. The right shoulder should stay on the floor. Repeat on the opposite side. Repeat this 10 times.

EMOTIONAL WELL-BEING
Today we would like you to focus on finding other ways to comfort yourself besides food. For instance you could phone a friend instead of reaching for a packet of crisps; you could watch your favourite video instead of sucking sweets; you could snack on fruit instead of chocolate; you could eat treats only when you have time to enjoy them; you could stop eating when you are full.

Healthy self-esteem can also motivate you to eat only things that are good for you. These self-esteem-boosting review tips may be helpful:

- Use affirmations: Whenever you hear the words 'I can't,' 'I won't,' 'I shouldn't,' 'I ought to' or 'What if ...?', replace them with positive ones: 'I can feel better,' 'I will feel confident,' 'There is nothing to fear,' 'I can handle it.'
- Confront your fear: The fear of doing something is often worse than the discomfort of doing it. If you are worried that PMS will destroy your health, take action to prevent that happening.
- Don't try to be perfect: Remind yourself that you have a right to be assertive, to have opinions and emotions and be successful. You also have the right to make mistakes and change your mind. There will be times when you won't eat healthily. It's not a big deal; just start eating healthily again tomorrow.
- Avoid unnecessary put-downs: If you have to be self-critical use self-respectful language and focus on your behaviour, NOT you as a person. For example, not 'I'm too fat for this dress,' but 'This dress isn't right for me, let me try another size.'
- Learn to respect the body you have, one day at a time. Women who respect their bodies and like themselves are irresistible and fun to be around, regardless of their dress size.
- Give yourself lots of non-food treats and pampering during stressful times. Have a massage or a facial, get your hair cut, visit old friends, go to the theatre, visit the seaside.
- Get support from people who enjoy your strengths and accept your weaknesses, not those who put you down.
- Be yourself, not someone else's idea of perfection. Keep an eye on your goals and make sure they are what you want.
- Give yourself time on your own and enjoy solitude and your own company and thoughts.
- Say 'no' more often. Tell yourself firmly, and often, that it is important to consider your own needs as well as other people's.

Day 4

NUTRITION

If you feel hungry all the time with smaller portion sizes, there are some tricks you can use to give you that full feeling:

- If you want to eat more, wait 10 minutes and see if you are still hungry. It takes longer than you think for your brain to register that your stomach is full.
- Keep a supply of healthy, low-fat snacks nearby for when you feel really hungry.
- Eat five small meals each day so you never get really hungry.
- Remember that it will take time for your stomach to adjust to smaller portion sizes. Give it a week or so.
- Drink a glass of water half an hour before you eat. You'll be less hungry and less tempted to overeat.
- If you are hungry, a useful tip from the Lighten Up team (see resources) is to smell your food first. 'Smell is the sense most directly related to the brain, and it's your sense of smell that will help you get back in touch with what your body needs,' says Lighten Up director Pete Cohen.

And when you do eat, take your time between mouthfuls and really savour what you are eating. Slow down. Make eating an event. You'll notice that you recognize when you are full sooner, and you'll also notice that you may be eating foods that you don't really enjoy.

EXERCISE

Do your 30-minute walk, your push-ups, oblique sit-ups and lunges (see below). Finish your routine with stretching. Remember, if it is the day of your class you don't need to do your walk, toning and stretching routine.

> **Lunges**
> Start by stepping forward making sure both feet point forward.
> Then slowly lunge forward over your front leg, bending at the
> knee. Return to standing and repeat with other leg. Repeat this 10
> times.

EMOTIONAL WELL-BEING

Now that you are aware of how food affects mood and that unhealthy
eating will make PMS symptoms worse and lead to weight gain you have
all the incentive you need to renew your motivation at this crucial five-
week stage to stick to the plan. If the going gets tough – and believe us it
will – never forget that by taking charge of your life and making positive
changes you are doing all you can to improve your health, beat PMS and
feel good about yourself.

Day 5

NUTRITION

Most nutritionists agree that eating little and often is the most effective
way to promote weight loss. So stick to five or six small meals and snacks
a day. Ideally breakfast and lunch should be your largest meals with a
light supper. Never skip meals, especially not breakfast, when you need
the energy most. Your brain needs a regular supply of glucose, so to keep
blood sugars stable develop a grazing mentality and eat little and often.
It's also a good idea to stop eating several hours before you go to bed, say
at around 8 p.m. This is because when you go to bed your body needs to
rest, not digest. The earlier in the day you eat, the more likely you are to
burn off calories even if you aren't particularly active that day.

Here are some weight-loss tips from women with PMS that you might find
helpful:

> *I had no idea that eating earlier in the day can actually be beneficial. I eat
> most of my food before 5 p.m. and just have a light snack in the evening. I*

wake up feeling so much better. I've got energy and my symptoms have virtually disappeared. **Amanda, 30**

I make sure that I allow myself two servings a day of sugar, for example two squares of chocolate or bread and jam. That way I don't feel so deprived. **Sarah, 28**

I have to eat out a lot, as it's part of my job. I now know that eating out doesn't have to be a problem if you just stick with the same healthy eating principles you apply at home. Ask for dressings on the side, look for grilled, poached, stir-fried or steamed dishes. Eat slowly and steer clear of the desert trolley, the bread basket, oily dressings, cream or cheese sauces and fried foods. **Rebecca, 36**

EXERCISE
Do your 30-minute walk, your sit-ups, push-ups, oblique sit-ups and lunges, and add alternate arm and leg raises (see below). Finish with your stretching routine.

> ### Alternate Arm/Leg Raises
> Lie down and keep your back as flat as you can. Slowly lift your right arm and leg. Lower and repeat with the left arm and leg. Repeat 10 times.

EMOTIONAL WELL-BEING
If thinking about food makes you feel anxious, one of the most thoroughly tested techniques is relaxation. Remember that high levels of anxiety are associated with high levels of stress hormones, and this won't help your PMS.

Slow down your breathing when you are craving food. The minute you become anxious your breathing becomes shallower and more rapid. To interrupt this, take slow, deep breaths through your nostrils and focus on your diaphragm as it moves up and down. As a rough guide, aim for four or five seconds to breathe in and the same for breathing out.

Meditation can also ease anxiety and stress according to many experts – perhaps because it shuts off your mind and allows your body to relax. Just sit upright, close your eyes and focus on your breathing. It might help to say a word such as 'calm', 'content' or 'peace' quietly to yourself. If unwanted thoughts about food intrude, simply notice them and then let them go, as if your thoughts are like a handful of sand that runs through your fingers. For the best results, aim to meditate for 10 to 20 minutes twice a day.

Day 6

NUTRITION

You may have noticed that when we talk of weight-loss we never mention calories or dieting. That's because calorie-counting and dieting take the focus away from nutrients. For example, one pack of chocolate biscuits can give you the calories you need for the day, but not the nutrients. So forget calorie-counting and dieting, and focus on getting all your essential nutrients instead. The more nutrient-rich your food, the more likely that symptoms will ease and the slimmer you will get. You won't feel hungry all the time, either.

EXERCISE

Do your 30-minute walk, all the toning exercises, and add some chair-dips (see below). Finish with your stretching routine.

Chair-dips
Find a strong chair and sit down. Now edge your bottom off the seat so your arms are holding your body weight. From here, slowly bend your elbows and lower your body until your upper arms are parallel to the ground, pushing up before repeating. Repeat 10 times.

EMOTIONAL WELL-BEING

The anxious/depressed state of mind that is typically part of PMS can result in feelings of worthlessness. You may feel that you can't handle things at certain times of the month, or make decisions. These insecure, negative feelings can add up over time and you may feel that you are losing your self-respect and your sense of being in control of your life.

Stop blaming yourself and try to see clearly the connections between your PMS and your mood. Your mood diary and symptom diary at the back of this book will help you with this. When you begin to associate the bad times with PMS, you can start to give yourself some room to breathe. You can leave the past behind and focus on the future. So today, *give yourself a break*. Allow yourself to leave behind guilt and self-doubt. Pamper yourself. Be kind, patient and generous with yourself.

Day 7

NUTRITION

Today we'd like you to re-read the good nutrition and weight-management information from Days 1 to 6 this week. You might want to jot down your own list of the main points and the reasons they are important. For example:

- watch my portion size – this can lead to weight gain which won't help my PMS
- watch my sugar intake –this can lead to weight gain and blood sugar problems – not good news for my PMS either
- eat little and often – this will keep my metabolic rate boosted and my blood sugar levels balanced
- eat a good breakfast – this will give me the energy I need at the start of the day
- how nutritious are my food choices? – To beat PMS and to control my weight, I need to make sure that my food choices are nutritious and so on …

And finally, bear in mind that you are designed to eat food that you can pull from the ground or pick off a tree. Have a look at your supermarket trolley this week when you go shopping. How much of the stuff in it grows on trees or can be pulled from the ground? If it's less than half the trolley, you need to have a rethink.

EXERCISE

Do your stretching routine today, but don't do any more than that. Ensure that you have a full day of rest and relaxation. You've earned it.

EMOTIONAL WELL-BEING

Today we would like you to re-read the emotional well-being notes way back in Week 3 about challenging negative thinking (pages 125–7). Just because you feel terrible does not mean you are terrible. Remind yourself to look for balance in every situation – nothing is totally bad. Remind yourself that the world does not revolve around you and your moods. Remember to assert your own needs. Stop exaggerating or thinking in all-or-nothing terms. And finally, rather than projecting your own feelings onto others, pay attention to your own feelings. Change your thoughts and you change your mood and your world.

VITALITY BOOSTER

This week's focus will be on techniques that you can learn and take with you anytime, anywhere to beat stress, improve mood and boost well-being. Identify those situations and people which trigger stress and consider trying to avoid them. If you can't avoid them, use some of the stress-busting techniques mentioned here.

> ### Basic Meditation Exercise
> Sit with an alert and relaxed posture so you feel comfortable. Keep your back straight and start to breathe steadily and deeply. Observe your breath as it flows in and out, feeling your stomach falling and rising. Give it your full attention. If you find your attention wandering, simply note the fact and gently bring your

thoughts back to your breath, to the rising and falling of your stomach. Try to do this for 5 to 10 minutes.

Don't immediately jump up afterwards. Bring yourself slowly back to consciousness. Become aware of the room around you, stretch and come back fully before you get up.

Basic Relaxation Exercise

Lie down in a peaceful room. Make sure you are comfortable and warm. Take 10 deep breaths and gently close your eyes. Now turn your attention to your head. Tense as hard as you can for a few seconds. Then let go suddenly. Your head is relaxed. Tense your face next – hold for a few seconds and relax. Continue in this way throughout your whole body – your neck, shoulders, down your arms, hand and fingers. Then back to your chest, stomach, hips, bottom, thighs, knees, feet and toes. Now check through your body. Are you still holding tension anywhere? If so, focus on that part.

Researchers believe that massage can help the brain to produce endorphins; the sense of well-being you feel from a massage can lower the amount of stress hormones in your body. Yoga, too, can be beneficial. MIND, the UK's mental health charity, recommends yoga as the single most effective stress-buster. Later in the plan we'll introduce you to some yoga exercises that can be used to reduce stress and boost well-being.

Instant Stress-busters

For you to use anytime, anywhere:

- Take deep breaths, jog on the spot, punch something like a cushion, or count to 10.
- Talk to friends, family, partners. If you don't feel you can talk to anyone, a trained counsellor may help you get in touch with your feelings and give you tips on how to deal with stress.
- Drink some kombucha tea, which contains B vitamins and other micronutrients and is made from a bacteria yeast culture.

- Homeopathic remedies that combat stress include Bryonia alba for anger, Lilium tigrinum for mood swings, and Belladona for restlessness and tearfulness.
- Kneel with your knees together and ankles relaxed. Allow your upper body to fall forward on to your legs so that your face is on the floor, arms by your sides. Relax.
- Fill out your personal space. Shrinking away from other people creates tension, so consciously relax your body, starting with the shoulders, and let yourself settle into your feet or your seat as if there were no one else around. Close your eyes or keep them slightly unfocused and turned downwards. Now imagine that you are expanding into the space just surrounding your body, flowing into it with every exhaling breath, taking more space for yourself.
- Put a few drops of Rescue Remedy – a preparation containing various flower essences – into a drink.
- Try the herbal remedy valerian for stress-related anxiety and insomnia. This sedative has been shown to help people fall asleep faster and to sleep better and longer without causing loss of concentration.
- Geranium, lavender and camomile are essential oils that can combat stress. Add a few drops to a warm bath or put a few drops in a burner or vaporizer to release the calming scents.
- Day-dreaming is a natural stress-busting technique. Allow your mind to wander for 4 minutes if you feel tense; maybe using your favourite picture or happy memory to help you drift off.
- Try this Ayurvedic technique for soothing the brain: for as long as possible, gently massage the point above your nose in the middle of your forehead in a very light circular movement.

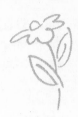

Week 6

Day 1

NUTRITION

Beating the Bloat
Enjoy eating your healthy menu today – and don't forget that
multivitamin and -mineral and calcium and magnesium supplement.
We'd also like to ask you something quite personal: Do you ever feel really
bloated when you are premenstrual?

> *I had to stop going to exercise classes in the week or so before my period. It*
> *was unpleasant for me – and for everyone else in the class. I thought I was*
> *doing all the right things, eating loads of fruit and veg and I'm vegetarian*
> *– but my stomach didn't agree. I had no idea that I was making the*
> *problem worse by eating my food too fast and eating gas-producing foods.*
> *I've changed my eating habits and never have to miss a class because of*
> *bloating and gas anymore.* **Mandy, 20**

The muscles in your intestine are very sensitive to oestrogen and
progesterone. This means that at different times in your cycle your

intestines may be slightly worse or slightly better at digesting your food. In the premenstrual period this can lead to an over-production of gas and that familiar bloated feeling.

If you suffer from premenstrual bloating, over-the-counter diuretics aren't a good idea as they leach valuable nutrients from you body. There are, however, a number of things you can do to help yourself. Some foods contain substances that are more gas-producing than others. The most common culprits are cabbage, cauliflower, broccoli, pulses such as baked beans, and lentils and chickpeas, so reduce your consumption if bloating and gas are a problem. Choose other vegetables such as spinach, carrots, mangetout, broad and French beans.

Resist drinking when you are eating. Try to leave half an hour after you have eaten before you have a drink, as by then your stomach will have more space available. Irregular eating habits can also increase bloating. If you don't eat regularly and leave your stomach empty for long periods, the secretion of digestive enzymes slows down. On the other hand, if you eat too much or eat too quickly this can overload your stomach, which can cause more gas. Also you tend to gulp more air when you eat quickly. So remember to eat small, regular meals and to eat them slowly.

Here's an anti-bloat sample menu to give you an idea of the kinds of foods to eat that can ease bloating. You might like to try it today or sometime this week.

Breakfast with multivitamin: Diluted fresh-pressed apple juice, poached egg on rye toast, 'live' natural yogurt sprinkled with nuts
Snack: Low-fat muffin with scraping of butter
Lunch: Steamed fish with mash and vegetables (carrots, broad beans and spinach); fruit salad with chopped almonds
Snack: Vegetable sticks with a teaspoon of peanut butter
Dinner: Carrot and orange soup, large salad with walnuts; baked apple with honey
You'll notice that we've included live yogurt. The reason is simple: put as much good bacteria as possible into your gut so that the bad gas-producing bacteria don't have the opportunity to grow. It's a good idea to

eat some 'live' yogurt containing the good bacteria – acidophilus and bifidus cultures – every day.

EXERCISE

Do your 30-minute walk, your toning exercises and your stretching routine today. Make sure that you stretch properly after toning and allow at least 30 seconds for each stretch. If this is the day of your class, remember you don't have to do your walk and toning session.

We'd also like to talk a little about yoga today and how helpful it can be if you have PMS.

Yoga, a Sanskrit word meaning 'union', originated in India more than 5,000 years ago. The practice of yoga is designed to quiet the mind by teaching you how to pay attention to your breathing and to the movement or stillness of your body.

Yoga postures re-establish structural integrity by stretching and strengthening muscles, expanding the natural range of motion, massaging internal organs, relaxing nerves and increasing blood circulation. And because yoga practice focuses and calms the mind, it can help ease feelings of anxiety, fatigue and depression, preventing or alleviating many stress-related conditions. If you do some yoga exercises in the morning you will have more energy to get through the day.

The most popular form of yoga in the West is called Hatha yoga, which focuses on the mind/body balance and uses physical postures, breathing techniques and meditation to restore the *prana* – the life-energy or vital force that flows through every living being. Since PMS is made worse by stress, tension and upset, the restorative effects of yoga may do much to ease your symptoms.

To learn more about yoga and find out how to choose a good instructor, see the Resources chapter. But if there just aren't enough hours in the day, starting tomorrow and for the rest of the week we are going to teach you some simple yoga exercises you can do by yourself at home. Even if you practise yoga for as little as 5 minutes a day, you can still experience many proven benefits.

EMOTIONAL WELL-BEING

Even when you are following this 12-week plan, it may still take two to three months for symptoms to ease. That's why it's a good idea to talk to your friends and family about your PMS. One of the best ways to help yourself is to share what you know.

> I was ashamed of my PMS. I was afraid I wouldn't be taken seriously at work. But when I started reading about PMS I discovered that other people were interested in hearing about it. For example, two new women joined me at work. They seemed nice at first and we worked well together, then suddenly they seemed to change. One got disinterested and the other bossy. I was practically in tears, thinking that I couldn't work with them. Two days later I found out that they both had just got their periods. Then I told them of something I just read. Women who spend a lot of time together often get their periods together. So that meant it might soon be all three of us PMSing together. We had a great laugh, which really cleared the air.
> **Mary, 34**

If you have a family, a partner or live with other people, you may need to point out what a nice person you are to live with most of the time. Ask them today if they will cut you some slack during PMS time. Have you put your PMS calendar on the wall with vulnerable days marked?

Day 2

NUTRITION

This week as you plan your menu, think about your salt intake. You may want to re-read the notes on cutting down on salt on pages 22–3.
The greater amount of sodium in your tissues, the greater the amount of water pulled into your tissues to balance it. So if you tend towards bloating, the more sodium you eat the worse the problem will get. Sodium, like sugar, lurks in almost everything you eat. Avoid foods

that are high in salt and try to eat those with a moderate to low sodium content.

High-sodium foods include: tinned meat or fish, baking soda, American, blue, Roquefort, cottage and parmesan cheese, chips, frozen dinners, meats (smoked, cured or pickled), commercially prepared pasta dishes, pickled vegetables, salty seasonings, tinned or packaged soups.

Medium-sodium foods include: baking powder, biscuits, muffins, bread, rolls, butter or margarine, cakes, pies, cereal, cheeses (other than those listed above), custard, gravy, ice-cream, mayonnaise, milk, mustard, nuts and seeds, peanut butter, frozen vegetables, soy sauce, tinned vegetables, yogurt.

Low-sodium foods include: low-sodium bread and crackers, shredded wheat, puffed wheat or rice, gruyere, ricotta, Swiss, unsalted or cream cheese, cream, eggs, flour, fruit juice, fruit, grains, fresh meat or fish, pasta, unsalted peanut butter, dried peas and beans, unsalted seasonings, fresh vegetables.

Like sugar, salt makes food taste nicer – but don't go overboard. Here are some review tips.

- Don't add salt to your food
- Only buy low-sodium tinned soup
- Don't buy foods that have been preserved with salt such as ham or sausage
- Avoid salty foods like crisps, crackers or salted nuts
- Avoid pickled foods like olives
- Don't use salty seasonings like MSG or soy sauce
- Limit your intake of baking soda and powder
- Cut the amount of salt you use in cooking down by half
- Throw away the salt cellar and use other seasonings to flavour your

food instead, such as cinnamon, lemon juice, basil, mint, nutmeg, rosemary, sage or thyme
- Increase your fluid intake. You need to drink more, not less, when you feel bloated. Increasing the amount you drink helps your body dilute the salt in your tissues and allows you to excrete more salt and fluid.
- Watch your caffeine intake. Although caffeine is a diuretic it won't ease the bloating because it also hinders the excretion of excess salt from your body.
- Eating more potassium-rich foods is a good way to bring down your body's sodium levels, as the two minerals balance each other out. Reach for the tomatoes, bananas, green leafy vegetables and fresh fruits.

EXERCISE
Do your 30-minute walk. Give yourself a day off from toning and stretching and try these yoga exercises instead.

Energizing Breath
When you are feeling stressed your breathing gets more shallow and rapid than usual. Your lungs are not fully expanded, so your body is rarely oxygenated fully. Just by taking a few deep breaths you can set yourself on the road to relaxation.

Stand with your feet together. Place your linked hands under your chin with your elbows together and lifted. Inhale slowly through your nose for a count of 5. As you do this, bring your elbows up as high as possible. Feel the breath at the back of your throat. Now gently let your head drop back and exhale completely through your mouth. At the end of the exhalation, slowly bring your elbows and palms together as your head returns to normal position. Try this 5 times today.

Mountain Pose

This yoga pose teaches correct posture and is the basis for all other standing poses.

Stand with your feet together so your big toes are touching and your heels are slightly apart. Let your arms relax by your sides. Spread and lengthen your toes, make sure your kneecaps are facing forward and keep your pelvis balanced over your legs. Now lengthen your spine. Continue to lengthen upwards, opening your chest. Drop your shoulders and lengthen the back of your neck. Hold this pose for 1 minute.

Sideways Stretch

Now stand straight with your legs 3 feet apart, your toes facing forward. Inhale and lift your right arm in the air. As you exhale, gently bend over to the left side, sliding your hand down your left leg. Don't strain, just go as far as you can with ease. Breathing normally, hold the position for a count of 5 or 10 if you feel strong enough. Inhale and return slowly to an upright position. Exhale, slowly lower your arm, and relax. Repeat the other side.

The Cat

On your hands and knees, as if you were a cat – weight distributed evenly between your palms and your knees, and your fingers pointing forward – as you slowly inhale pull your stomach muscles tight and curve your back towards the ceiling, like a cat arching its back. Tuck your chin into your chest to complete the cat-like pose and hold for a count of 5. Then relax the spine and bring your head back to its normal position as you slowly exhale. Continue exhaling as you reverse the arch of your spine, pulling your head back and lifting your bottom in the air. Inhale as you move back to your starting position. Continue inhaling as you repeat the exercise, first arching like a cat then exhaling as you pull your head, neck and spine backward. Do the exercise slowly and never rush.

> **Pose of a Child**
>
> This is a good one to do at the end of a yoga session to ease your
> body into a totally relaxed state.
>
> Tuck your legs underneath you as you sit on a mat with your heels
> directly underneath your bottom and your knees pointing forward.
> Place your knees apart about 10 inches while keeping your toes
> together, forming a V with your thighs. Roll your upper body
> forward to the floor with your arms extended loosely in front of
> you. Your forehead should touch the floor if possible. Keep your
> bottom in contact with your heels. Relax in this position for a
> count of 20 or as long as you like. Slowly roll back to a sitting
> position.

EMOTIONAL WELL-BEING

Today we would like you to do a bit more advance planning if you think
physical discomfort and mood problems are going to affect you. Here are a
few things you can do:

- Schedule fewer activities (perhaps only the necessary ones) on the
  days you suspect symptoms will be most severe. Make yourself less
  busy and plan to devote more time to pampering yourself or doing
  something that makes you feel more in control: a bubble bath,
  spending time alone, listening to music, reading?
- On PMS days, figure out what you want or need and post a list of it
  somewhere visible, like the fridge, for everyone to see. For example 1) I
  need to finish x report at work 2) I need to go to my yoga class 3) I
  need to make my own dinner today and nobody else's 4) I need to tidy
  my room today. You may find that the people in your life take to this
  list-posting with ease. Now they know what to expect, they aren't
  going to be alarmed or surprised if you keep yourself to yourself.

Day 3

NUTRITION

Food Intolerances
Some women experience stomach pains, bloating and flatulence after eating certain foods.

Food intolerances interfere with digestion and therefore make bloating worse. Food intolerances can develop suddenly, or you could be intolerant to foods that you tend to eat most often. It isn't always the case that you naturally dislike a food you shouldn't have.

It is important to understand the difference between an allergy and a food intolerance. The term food intolerance is used when a specific food or food ingredient causes an unpleasant reaction such as digestive problems, bloating or fatigue. A food allergy is a disorder of the immune system aggravated by certain foods – peanuts and shellfish are the worst offenders – which creates an allergic rash or reaction.

If you suspect that you have a food intolerance, you can make adjustments to your diet and get on with your life. The difficult part is finding out what you are sensitive to – it might be a good idea to seek the advice of a doctor or nutritionist before starting your investigation. Remove the suspected item from your diet for one week. Make sure that your body is not going to become malnourished by replacing it. (For the next few days we will discuss the most common food intolerances and how to find nutritious replacements.) If your symptoms disappear, you can assume they were related to that food. If they continue you should seek professional advice, as once you start removing more than one food from your diet, things can get complicated.

EXERCISE
Do your 30-minute walk, your toning and your stretching – and make sure your stretching routine includes the yoga poses below.

Standing Forward Bend

Start with the Energizing Breath and then the Mountain Pose (see page 183) From the Mountain Pose go into this Standing Forward Bend, which will release and invigorate you.

Stand 1 foot away from a wall with your feet hip-width apart and your back to the wall. Place your hands on the wall and rest your buttocks against it. Now place your hands on your hips and inhale. Exhale slowly and bend forward from the hips. Bend your arms and clasp your elbows. Relax your neck and head as well as your throat and eyes. Hold for 30 seconds. Release your arms slowly, inhale and return to the Mountain Pose.

Sideways Stretch

Stand straight with your legs 3 feet apart with your toes facing forwards. Inhale deeply and lift your right hand in the air. As you exhale, gently bend over the left side, sliding your left hand down your left leg. Don't strain, just go as far as you can with ease. Hold the position for a count of 5 or 10. Inhale and slowly return to an upright position. Exhale slowly, lower your arm and relax. Repeat on the other side, then repeat the whole movement.

EMOTIONAL WELL-BEING

Today our advice sounds simple: Accept support. You have to remember, however, that it's not someone else's responsibility to remember to give you support. You may have to ask for it.

Only you know what you are feeling, but people who love or care about you do want to help. We may not always know exactly what we need. We may have to tell our loved ones that all we want is their understanding, that we value their support and love and that when PMS strikes they need to show us even more. This is sharing your feelings in a positive way. You are involving your friends and family without wallowing in self-pity. So allow others to help, ask for their help, and take it when it is offered.

Day 4

NUTRITION

Some scientists believe that half the world's population is unable to tolerate cow's milk. Lactose is the natural sugar found in all animal milk products, and people who are lactose intolerant have problems breaking it down, leading to a build-up of undigested lactose in the gut and resulting in digestive problems, bloating, gas and fatigue.

If you suspect that you are lactose-intolerant, today we are going to suggest PMS-friendly alternatives. These will help replace the calcium that you lose if you are sensitive to milk.

Especially if you can't tolerate milk, supplement your diet with a bone formula containing both calcium and magnesium in a ratio of 2:1 – two tablets a day. Do make sure, though, that your supplement isn't derived from lactose.

Many foods contain calcium, including sesame seeds, leafy green vegetables, brazil nuts, almonds, tinned salmon, watercress, figs, broccoli and seaweed. However, none of these is as rich in calcium as dairy produce.

The problem of osteoporosis is a serious one, and it appears that women with PMS may be more prone, so if you are lactose-intolerant it is crucial that you don't neglect your calcium intake.

Soya milk, cheese and yogurt can be safely eaten. If you are intolerant just to cow's milk protein, as many women are, you can also enjoy goat's and sheep's milk. You can make your own milk-free cakes and biscuits by replacing the butter with milk-free margarine. Instead of cream or yogurt on your fruit desserts, make a fruit coulis as a sauce. And Chinese, Thai, Indian and Malaysian food uses little or no milk produce, so these are good choices when eating out.

EXERCISE

Do your 30-minute walk and your stretching routine. Practise the yoga posture below and have a go again first thing tomorrow when you get out of bed.

> ### *Head-to-Knee Posture*
> Start with your Energizing Breath and Mountain Pose.
>
> Inhale and lift your arms above your head. Place your palms together and stretch your body upwards. (This is great for realigning the spine and releasing tension.) As you lower your arms, exhale slowly through your nose. Repeat the movement.
>
> Now place your left foot about 3 feet in front of your right. Inhale and lift your arms above your head, palms together. As you exhale – with your head up, back flat and legs straight – bend forwards aiming your hands just past your knee. Don't strain. Relax in your maximum position for 5 seconds, breathing normally.
>
> Inhale and lift your head, slowly returning to the upright position. Then exhale, lowering your arms as you do, and relax.
>
> Repeat on the other side, placing your right foot 3 feet in front of your left.

EMOTIONAL WELL-BEING

Today we would like you to re-read the emotional well-being notes for Week 4 on dealing with anger and depression. If things start to get to you this week, try the RETHINK technique discussed there.

Day 5

NUTRITION

Some women feel less bloated and have fewer problems with digestion, and more energy, when they avoid wheat and gluten foods.

The first step is to establish whether you are sensitive to wheat or to gluten.

Wheat is a grain, whereas gluten is a protein found in wheat, oat, rye and barley. If you are just sensitive to wheat you can eat oats, rye and barley. However, if you are sensitive to gluten you need to avoid all these grains and the products containing them – including beer and whisky. You also need to avoid food starch and bread, crackers, biscuits, cakes and other products containing flour.

The Coeliac Society (see the Resources chapter for the address) produces a list of products that are gluten-free; you may want to have this as your source of reference.

The best thing to do is not to focus on the foods you *can't* have but to think about all the foods that naturally don't contain gluten and how you can use them to make exciting dishes. For example, rice, risotto, potato bakes, buckwheat pancakes, sauces or pies using potato flour or cornflower. It's just a matter of changing your mindset – which, like beating PMS, takes time and effort. Once you've managed it, however, a gluten-free or wheat-free diet can be just as delicious and varied as any other healthy eating plan.

EXERCISE

Did you do the Head-to-Knee yoga posture this morning? How did it feel? Do your toning, your 30-minute walk and your stretching routine. And make sure you know how to do the yoga pose below so you can start your day with it tomorrow.

> ***Forwards and Backwards Bend***
> Do your Energizing Breath and Mountain Pose.
>
> Inhale and slowly stretch your arms above your head. Exhale slowly through your nose as you bend forwards, keeping your back flat and legs straight until you reach your maximum without straining. Stay there for a count of 5 or 10, breathing normally. You may not be able to reach far to start with, but one day your chin will be on your shins if you keep practising. Inhale and come up slowly into an upright position, hands stretched above your head. Bend backward, looking at your thumbs and exhaling in your maximum position. Breathing normally hold for a count of 5, inhale and return to an upright position. Exhale, lower your arms and relax. Repeat.

EMOTIONAL WELL-BEING

If you find it extremely hard to share your concerns and ask support from the people in your life, you might benefit from talking to a counsellor. Almost everyone can use this kind of support from time to time. It's important to make sure that the person you see has the specialist training needed and is well informed about women's issues and health concerns. Ask your GP for advice, or take a look at the Resources chapter for the address of counselling organizations that can send you information about qualified counsellors in your area.

Day 6

NUTRITION

Try putting your fork and knife down between bites, and really take the time to chew your food properly today. Eating on the run tends to lead to digestive troubles which can just make symptoms of PMS seem even worse. So sit down when you eat your healthy menu, and take your time.

Some people find that certain additives upset their stomachs and cause mood swings and depression. The most common culprits are sulphur dioxide, sodium metabisulphite and potassium metabisulphite (used as preservatives), yellow azo dyes and monosodium glutamate. If you suspect you have an additive insensitivity, you just need to check labels. This does take time, but you will soon know which foods you can and cannot enjoy.

EXERCISE
Do your 30-minute walk, remembering to keep your pace brisk. Do your stretching routine and have a go at the Rishis posture, below.

Do your Energizing Breath and Mountain Pose.

Rishis Posture
Stand with your legs about 3 feet apart. Inhale and gently stretch your arms into the air. As you exhale, bend forwards slowly and, with your legs straight and back flat, grasp your left leg with your right hand. Don't strain, just grasp wherever is comfortable. Slowly lift your left arm and turn your body so you are facing your left hand. Hold for a count of 5 or 10. Then slowly lower your arm and relax forwards, clasping your legs and gently pulling your body towards them.

Inhale and, as you exhale, repeat the movement on the other side, raising your right arm. Relax forwards, clasping both legs drawing your body inwards.

Inhale and return to upright, stretching your arms above your head. Put your hands on your waist with thumbs in front and fingers behind. Now gently bend back, exhaling as you reach your maximum bend. Hold for 5. Inhale and return to upright. Exhale. Relax and repeat.

Before you go to bed tonight, take this book upstairs with you and remind yourself to look at it first thing.

EMOTIONAL WELL-BEING
Think about your support group today. It doesn't have to be large – you and one other person will do. Mothers can be a source of comfort and advice. Female friends can also be a great support, especially if they have PMS themselves. Your partner may also be a reassuring presence, rubbing your back or tummy to make you feel good about yourself.

Day 7

NUTRITION
Do your shopping list this weekend and your weekly shop. Don't forget that multivitamin and -mineral and your calcium and magnesium, and when you plan your healthy menu today include a small food treat. Perhaps you could eat out today or have a slice of chocolate cake. Whatever your treat is, enjoy it!

EXERCISE
Good morning!

Instead of your walk, toning and stretching, today we'd like you to do all the yoga poses we have introduced you to this week in one 30-minute session. You may want to do it now, first thing, or later in the day when you feel more awake.

After your session, think about how you feel. Is yoga an exercise option you would like to explore further? If it is, you could think of joining a class or buying a self-help book or video so that you can learn many more poses and discover their incredible health benefits.

EMOTIONAL WELL-BEING
If you haven't got an informal support group and counselling doesn't appeal, you may want to consider joining a formal support group. If you

live in a big city you may be able to locate one through a university medical centre or PMS clinic. You could also ask your GP to give you a referral to a group. A support group may be your main resource for help and comfort, and we've listed several for you to get in touch with in the Resources chapter.

If you can't find a support group in your area, you may want to start one yourself. If you can get two or three women with PMS together on a regular basis, you have your group. Be sure to keep the discussion upbeat, focusing on remedies that have helped. If you find advice on the Internet, be sure to remember that what you are reading may be only one person's opinion and not a treatment that has been based on scientific research, like this book.

VITALITY BOOSTER

Enjoying Your Social Life

Study after study[1] has shown that social contact can increase happiness and feelings of health and well-being. People with social lives feel supported, part of a network, have fewer colds and flu and feel more positive about life. So this week, have a think about the following:

- What is your social life like? Are you spending time with people who make you feel good about yourself? What would you like to do more of? Whom would you like to see more of? Perhaps you would like to meet more people, or perhaps you would like to spend more time with your family?
- Have you thought of visiting your neigbour? A shocking number of people have never even spoken to their neighbours. Why not introduce yourself and invite your neighbour over for a coffee?
- Share yourself. Don't hold your feelings, thoughts and dreams inside. Share them with friends and family. People who hold things inside tend to feel isolated, and that others do not understand them. Studies[2] show that those who share feel more supported and more content even when things don't go their way.

- Have you thought of volunteer work? Studies[3] show that people who
  volunteer their time to help others have a sense of purpose, feel
  appreciated and are less likely to feel unhappy about their lives. Giving
  even an hour a month will be good for your health, too.

Week 7

Day 1

NUTRITION

Time to Re-assess
Today we'd like you to go back to Week 1 of the plan and refresh your memory on all the nutrition information there. Are you making sure you're getting enough magnesium in your diet? Now that you are six weeks into the plan, how much of the advice given are you incorporating into your daily meals and snacks? Do you need to make any changes? Or are you doing just fine? Are you remembering to take your multivitamin and -mineral and calcium and magnesium supplements every day?

EXERCISE

Get Active!
The health of animals tends to suffer when they are confined in small places, so it's hardly surprising that our health suffers too when we get too sedentary. To be healthy you should be active outside your work-out,

too. Your 30-minute walk will certainly improve your fitness, but if that is all you do for the whole day your activity levels may still be too low.

Three or four minutes of brisk marching in place and you will have taken steps towards a healthy body simply by getting up when the adverts are on. In the office do the same when waiting for a fax to arrive, the photocopier to switch on or the kettle to boil. Take five minutes of every hour to jog on the spot or walk briskly round the room. When you are doing errands, park the car away from the shop, and use the stairs instead of a lift. If you are worried about what friends and family and co-workers will think when they see you dancing around, just tell them it's doctor's orders. Movement is your birthright. Make sure you claim it today.

EMOTIONAL WELL-BEING

Your PMS Charts

Today we would like you to take a look at your getting to know your own PMS charts. As you glance at the last six weeks' worth of charts, ask yourself:

- Is there a pattern to my symptoms?
- Do things seem easier to handle now I know when to expect my symptoms?
- Am I feeling a difference in my outlook after following the plan?

If you do feel more positive, give yourself a pat on the back. If you don't feel much better, remind yourself that it can take up to two or three months to feel the benefits. Hang in there. Don't give up now – you are already past the halfway mark.

Day 2

NUTRITION

Check-up Time!

Have a look at Week 2 of the plan today and re-read all the information on nutrition for that week. Are you getting enough calcium and magnesium in your diet? Ask yourself how well you are sticking to the guidelines.

EXERCISE

Crank Up a Notch

Do your usual 30-minute walk and stretching today. If you have been walking on a regular basis over the past few weeks, you might want to take it further and partake in more vigorous activity. If, however, you enjoy what you are doing and don't feel ready to go up a gear yet, carry on with your brisk walking. There is plenty of time later to expand your workout. The ideal would be to combine five or six periods of moderate activity (e.g. your 30-minute walk and toning and stretching) with one or two periods of more vigorous activity a week. A combination of moderate and vigorous activity adds variety and interest to your exercise routine.

To ensure that you do vigorous exercise safely, first check with your GP that it is safe for you to do. Do not exercise vigorously if you feel unwell or are recovering from a viral illness such as a cold or flu, or if you have been taking painkillers. Then work out your maximum heart rate for aerobic exercise. To do this you have to subtract your age in years from the heart rate of 220 beats per minute e.g. 220 – 40 = 180 beats per minute. This gives you the maximum heart rate in beats per minute for aerobic exercise, which increases your heart fitness. Now measure your actual heart rate during exercise by taking your pulse at your neck or wrist. Count the number of beats per minute (or per 15 seconds and then multiply by four). Stop straightaway if you ever experience pain in the chest, neck or upper left arm, joint pain, dizziness or faintness, severe breathlessness or exhaustion.

To start with you should exercise to 50 per cent of your maximum heart rate. Moderate activity (brisk walking and gentle jogging) is 40 – 60 per cent, vigorous activity is 60 – 80 per cent (more intense jogging or running). Try to do 20 minutes of moderate to vigorous activity once or twice a week.

EMOTIONAL WELL-BEING

How Are Your Mood Swings?

Take some time today to re-read your mood diary that you started way back in Week 1. Has tracking your moods helped you see when mood swings and feelings of sadness relates to PMS and when they don't? If you think they are PMS-related, remind yourself that by the end of the 12-week plan these should ease. If they are not PMS-related, remind yourself that even though the plan can't solve all your problems, it can help you feel more in control of your life. And when you feel in control you are better able to face challenges.

Day 3

NUTRITION

Look Back at Week 3

We'd like you to re-read the nutrition notes for Week 3 of the plan today. Have you incorporated the advice into your daily menus today? Don't worry if you haven't. Just make sure that over the next five weeks you eat healthily every day. If you want to beat PMS, you need to put the effort in now.

EXERCISE

How Vigorous Are You?

Try to do a 10-minute moderate activity warm-up today, and then 20 minutes of more vigorous activity. Cool down with your stretching routine. Write down how you feel before and after your more vigorous exercise session. We suspect that you may feel a little reluctant before, but you'll feel terrific afterwards. There is nothing like vigorous exercise to energize and invigorate.

EMOTIONAL WELL-BEING

Feeling Happy
What does leading a fulfilling life mean? It doesn't mean being happy all the time, but it does signify having the ability to cope with life's ups and downs. It means gaining a sense of achievement from small pleasures, from planting a few bulbs on a grey afternoon to writing a difficult letter. It means finding equilibrium within yourself and balancing your emotions. It is also about coping with and welcoming change; acknowledging that life is a process and that we need to be flexible in mind and body and spirit.

Psychologists have been researching what makes people happy and have found that fame and fortune are not the answer. Rather, as psychologist David G Myers wrote in a (July/August) 1993 article for *Psychology Today*, 'Happiness is less a matter of what we want than wanting what we have.'

Happiness is about living in the now, rather than worrying about the future. It is about savouring every precious moment, the first stretch as you wake up, the first daffodil's appearance after a long winter, a letter from an old friend, a hug from your child. Pascal had some wise words: 'So we never live, but we hope to live – and as we are always preparing to be happy, it is inevitable we should never be so.' Are you hoping to live, or are you already living?

Day 4

NUTRITION

Re-focus on Week 4
Turn to Week 4 of the plan today and re-read the good nutrition section. Take notes to remind yourself of the important points.

EXERCISE

Family Fitness

Do your 30-minute walk, your toning and your stretching today. Have a think, too, about how fit your family and friends are. You getting fit will inspire the people close to you to get off their backsides, too, and take better care of themselves.

If you are a mum, encourage your kids to exercise. Play sports with your children or join them on their roller-blades in the park. Make family holidays rambling, trekking, and climbing ones, for example.

If you are in a relationship, your partner will benefit, too. Don't let the significant others in your life settle for a potbelly. Encourage them to work out with you.

EMOTIONAL WELL-BEING

Think Positive!

Re-read the notes on positive thinking on pages 111–12. Remind yourself that research shows that people who are most satisfied with their lives have self-esteem and a sense of optimism. Learn to like yourself a bit more. List your good points. List your achievements, great and small. Separate your feelings of self-worth from others or from status symbols such as a job, a car or your children's exam results. You are a separate person with your own unique needs and talents. Recognize what and who affects your sense of self-esteem, and challenge negative thinking in every way you can.

Day 5

NUTRITION

Refresh Your Memory of Week 5

Have a look at Week 5 of the plan today and re-read the nutritional

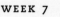

information there. You may like to take some notes to refresh your memory on the important points.

EXERCISE

Cycle Sense

Do your stretching followed by your 10-minute warm-up and walk, and then, if you feel up to it, launch into your choice of more vigorous activity (if you don't, just keep on walking). Cycling is a good option if you are overweight and are discouraged by the initial discomfort of jogging or walking. Cycling is non-weight bearing and is less likely to damage your joints than running. If you are cycling outside make sure you wear a helmet and make sure, too, that you choose the right bike for your build. Get the right clothes, too – not necessarily lycra shorts. You need clothes that can keep out the rain and cover you up if you feel cold and stiff.

EMOTIONAL WELL-BEING

Be Kind!

Today we would like you to re-read the notes on managing your emotions on pages 123–4. Remind yourself to be kinder to yourself and accept that you have your own needs and desires. Remind yourself that acknowledging your emotions is essential for good emotional – and physical – health.

Day 6

NUTRITION

Update on Week 6

Today we would like you to go back to last week's nutrition information and re-read it.

EXERCISE

Housework Boosters

Do your 30-minute walk, your toning and stretching routines today. And if you have housework to do today, think of this as a way to polish off the pounds. Slow your movements down and focus on muscle control to tone your muscles:

- Instead of bending to pick things up or to load and unload the washing machine or dishwasher, use squats to tone your bottom and thighs.
- Work trunk twists and turns into wiping surfaces, and arm flexes into dusting and window-cleaning.
- Lunges and leg raises to the side while vacuuming can tone your inner thighs and calves.
- A bit of carpet-beating, scrubbing and running up and down stairs will do wonders for weight-management.
- Do sit-ups when you feel exhausted at the end of your housework session and are waiting for the kettle to boil.

EMOTIONAL WELL-BEING

Mind and Body Harmony

Remind yourself today of the strong links between your mind and your body. Recognize your less-than-healthy attitudes to food, body-image or ageing. Remind yourself that you have the power to choose healthier and more effective ways to live, and that the 12-week plan is helping you make these changes.

Day 7

NUTRITION

Tweak Your Menus

This week has been a refresher week as we've looked at all the nutrition information from the first six weeks of the plan. Do you need to make any changes to your daily food intake, or are you doing OK? Was there anything important that you needed reminding about? Renew your commitment to yourself to stick with the plan over the next five weeks, and to make changes if changes need to be made.

EXERCISE

Enjoy Yourself, Assess Yourself

How about an early morning yoga session at home? Or perhaps you would just like to take a walk in the park today? Whatever you decide, make sure your exercise session today is gentle and relaxing.

Review the last seven weeks of your exercise routine. How have you done? Today is the day to let go of any excuses that have until now stopped you benefiting from the joy of being active:

- *I'm too tired.* In fact, being more active raises your energy level. If you find it hard to exercise after work, try to do your activity session when your energy level is highest — first thing in the morning or in your lunch hour.
- *I look fat in my leotard/swimsuit.* You don't have to wear a leotard at your local gym. Many gyms have women-only times and have T-shirt-only policies. A T-shirt and leggings or baggy bottoms are just as trendy.
- *I don't have time.* Taking regular exercise can be built into your daily life. You can walk or cycle instead of using the bus or car. You can use the stairs instead of the lift. Even housework can help.
- *I can't afford it.* Walking is great and it's free.
- *I have back pain/leg pain.* Regular exercise will help strengthen the muscles that support your back and legs. Swimming and cycling are excellent for joint pain. Seek advice from your GP on what exercises you can do.

Make a commitment to yourself now to include exercise in your life on a daily basis. Starting today, at the back of your mood diary keep a record of your daily workout sessions to monitor your progress.

EMOTIONAL WELL-BEING

Celebrate Friendship

Today, call, write or send an e-mail to a good friend. It is surprising how many women don't keep in touch with their friends as much as they like with jobs, families, partners, kids, pets, housework, shopping and chores always higher on their list of priorities. So today, for however much time you can spare, spend it talking to or writing to a friend you trust and care about.

VITALITY BOOSTER

Laugh More

This week's focus is all about bringing more laughter into your life.

In September 1991, Robert Holden, founder of the Happiness Project and the Coaching Success Partnership, a leading-edge consultancy working with individuals and groups worldwide, opened the doors to Britain's first official NHS Laughter Clinic. Holden's Laughter Clinic is perhaps best described as 'a support group for joy' and thousands of doctors, nurses and therapists have attended Laughter Clinic workshops over the past 10 years.

Intuitively, we know that laughter is good for us. Think for a moment how your body feels whenever you laugh or smile – words like 'relaxed', 'warm', 'whole', 'free' and 'light-hearted' often come to mind. Trust your intuition! Laughter, happiness and a joyful heart really do offer a medicinal, therapeutic touch.

A Work-out

It is possible for all 400 muscles of the body to move during laughter – thus laughter has been playfully labelled by some as a form of 'internal aerobics'. If you were able to sustain a belly laugh for one full hour, you could laugh off as many as 500 calories! Medical research also shows that whenever we laugh we release a wave of chemicals through the body including the endorphin hormone, which is also released during healthy exercise. Endorphins (their name means 'of morphine') are the body's natural pain-relaxers – they stimulate feelings of well-being and joy. One of the mottoes of The Laughter Clinic Project is, 'If you are too busy to laugh, you are too busy!'

HAPPY CELL

The research of Dr Lee Berk at Loma Linda University School of Medicine, California, shows that laughter, happiness and joy 'inspire' the immune system to create white 'T' cells, commonly called 'happy cells', which help to prevent infection. Dr Berk's research has also found that the 'mirthful laughter experience', as he calls it, appears to reduce serum levels of cortisol, dopac, adrenaline and growth hormone, thereby creating the reverse of the stress response. Both physically and psychologically, it is as if laughter acts as a 'safety valve' for the discharge of nervous energy.

The following five prescriptions are recommended by Dr Robert Holden from his happiness project website (www.happiness.co.uk):

1 **S** is for **Smile**. Make an effort to be more friendly today, just for the fun of it. In a study[1] of adults of various ages, a tendency was found to mimic the expression of those around them. Sad faces evoked sad faces, and smiling faces evoked smiles and happiness.
2 **M** is for **Make**. Don't wait for happiness to happen, *make* it happen. Some pursue happiness – others create it!
3 **I** is for **Impulse**, **Innovation** and the **Irregular**. Change a perception, alter a belief, entertain a new thought, communicate differently, act adventurously.
4 **L** is for the greatest dose of medicine of all: **Love**. Let someone know that you love them today.
5 **E** is for **Enjoyment**. When was the last time you went out to play? Indulge yourself, invest in yourself, give yourself something to smile about.

Week 8

Day 1

NUTRITION

Eating to Boost Energy
Enjoy your healthy meals this week, and don't forget your multivitamin and -mineral, calcium and magnesium supplements every day.

This week we are going to think about ways to beat the feelings of listlessness and fatigue that often accompany PMS. We'll start today by looking at the amount of iron in your diet.

Do you drink a lot of tea? Do you avoid red meat? Do you get heavy periods? These three things combined can contribute to anaemia. Anaemia is a lack of haemoglobin – the red blood cells that help carry oxygen around your body. If the oxygen capacity in your blood is reduced, your muscles won't get the oxygen they need and you will feel tired most of the time.

There are several sorts of anaemia, but the most common is iron-deficiency anaemia. Red meat is a major source of iron, while the tannin in tea can leach away iron supplies, as can heavy periods. Symptoms of iron deficiency include pale skin and dark circles under your eyes. You may also get frequent mouth ulcers, a sore tongue and split or brittle nails. Concentration is often poor and fatigue is a real problem all month long.

If you think you have anaemia, see your doctor first, as a blood test can check your iron levels. The obvious answer would be to take iron supplements, but some health experts believe that iron contributes to the build-up of toxins in your body. Whether this is true or not has yet to be concluded, but iron supplements can cause constipation, so on the whole it is best to try and make sure you get your iron from the foods that you eat rather than from supplements. If you do take iron supplements only do so for a short period – say three months – and make sure you keep checking your iron levels with your doctor, or take a natural iron tonic such as floravital. Take low-dose iron supplements (no more than 15 mg, as more can be toxic and cause constipation) and take with vitamin C and B to increase absorption.

If you are a vegetarian you might want to take kelp supplements. Wheatgerm, dried fruit, shellfish, sardines and egg yolk are also sources of iron, as are red and dark green fruits and veg.

To boost your iron levels this week, why not sprinkle some wheatgerm on your yogurt, snack on dried fruit or enjoy sardines or scrambled eggs on toast? If you are not a vegetarian, allow yourself to have a small portion of red meat once a week. If you are a vegetarian, snack on apricots or a small bar of dark, organic chocolate, and make sure your soya milk and cereals are iron fortified. Finally, think about replacing tea with herbal drinks that don't contain caffeine or tannin, or at least cut back on the amount of tea you drink. You may want to refer back to our cut-back-on-caffeine survival tips on page 56.

EXERCISE

If listlessness and fatigue are a problem, even though it is the last thing you may feel like doing, regular exercise really can give you more energy.

Moving, stretching and toning all help to convert your food into energy by bringing more oxygen to your cells. Exercise also boosts your circulation and helps your lymphatic system, which in turn aids the detoxification process of your body.

EMOTIONAL WELL-BEING
An often-neglected cause of fatigue is feeling low or depressed. Remember, if low moods only occur in the week or so before your period they are related to your PMS, but if they appear all month long there may be another cause.

Signs of depression include:

- loss of joy in life and interest in friends and family
- loss of interest in other people and difficulty relating to others
- low self-esteem
- feelings of hopelessness and feeling that nothing can be done to improve your life
- low motivation levels
- lack of appetite, unexplained aches and pains, sleep disturbances and lack of energy.

If you think you may be suffering from depression, re-read the notes on dealing with it on page 299. The next step is to see your doctor, who may refer you to a therapist or counsellor. Your emotions diary can be a useful form of therapy to release feelings of pain and sadness. Spend 10 or so minutes a day writing down your feelings. Remember that stored anger, grief and sadness can be depleting. Talking over your problems with someone you trust can help.

Day 2

NUTRITION

Go Green!
Today we'd like to remind you of the importance of including lots of green leafy vegetables in your diet, such as spinach, watercress, kale and broccoli, and sufficient fruit such as citrus fruits and berries. The vitamin C found in fruit and green leafy vegetables also helps to increase the absorption of iron. When cooking vegetables, try not to over-boil them as this can reduce their iron content by up to 20 per cent.

Today, before you eat your meal, have a look at your plate. Divide up the meal and make sure that half of it is vegetables, a quarter protein and the rest carbohydrates. Meals in this kind of proportion can work wonders for boosting energy, losing weight and beating PMS.

EXERCISE

Instant Pick-Me-Up Routine
Do your 10-minute warm-up followed by 20 minutes of vigorous exercise today. If you sometimes find it difficult to exercise because you feel so tired, remind yourself that beating fatigue and PMS involves long-term lifestyle changes. You won't rediscover your energy overnight; it takes two to three months, but every time you exercise you take one more step towards better health.

Try this instant pick-me-up first thing in the morning or if you have been sitting down for a long time. It pumps fresh air into your body.

Stand upright and check your posture (see pages 154–7 if you need help with this). Breathe in, lift your arms up over your head and stretch as high as you can. Slowly breathe out as you take your arms down again behind your head and circle them towards your hips. Do this three more times. You need to make big circles with your arms. Now do this in the other direction four times.

To finish, stretch up, take a deep breath and let your body flop forwards with your knees bent. As you swing down, breathe out, pushing every last bit of air out of your body and saying 'aaaa' out loud to help you do this. Then slowly come up, breathing in again.

EMOTIONAL WELL-BEING

Never Say Never
Life is often full of challenges that can drain your energy levels. But you can drain your own confidence and energy without realizing it by thinking 'I can't' or ' I won't be able to.' If you find yourself saying these today, stop and take a moment to reflect. You can rise to whatever challenge is being presented, so think along more positive lines and switch to phrases such as 'I can' and 'I will.' You'll notice an immediate boost in your energy levels.

Day 3

NUTRITION

Get Fresh
Certain foods can boost your energy levels and others can deplete them. For practitioners of yoga, the energy of a food is known as its *prana* (*prana* is Sanskrit for 'life-force'). Foods high in *prana* include fresh wholefoods, preferably in season and easy to cook and digest. The more a food is tampered with, the more nutrients it loses, so try to eat whole foods that are as fresh as possible.

Protein is an important energy source, so try not to neglect your protein intake. US nutritionist Dr Barry Spears offers convincing evidence in his *Zone* books that a diet sufficient in protein gives us more energy, whereas a diet too high in carbohydrate leads to fatigue. Many women in a misguided attempt to lose weight cut down too drastically on their protein and fat and eat way too much carbohydrate.

By eating a diet of about 25 per cent low-fat protein and by making sure that you never eat a carbohydrate snack unless it is combined with some form of protein, you can increase your energy levels and promote weight loss.

EATING-FOR-ENERGY TIPS

- Whenever possible, eat food that is unprocessed. Pesticides, hormones and additives rob food of its energy potential.
- Avoid processed margarines. They contain transfatty acids, which make margarine spreadable but are hard for your body to process. A small amount of butter is actually healthier than an artificial spread.
- Cut out sugar and keep your tea, coffee and alcohol intake moderate, as all these will interfere with blood sugar levels.
- Don't re-heat, overcook or store food for too long – you can't afford to lose those nutrients.
- Make sure you drink enough water throughout the day – if you don't you will feel very tired. Water is an essential and often forgotten nutrient and, like a houseplant, you need a constant supply.
- Chew your food thoroughly. Your saliva contains an enzyme that helps to pre-digest your food so you can absorb it better.
- Ensure that you include sufficient high-quality, low-fat protein in your diet.

EXERCISE

Breathing for a Boost

Do your 30-minute walk, your toning and your stretching today, and try the following yoga breathing exercises designed to increase energy when you feel in need of a quick lift.

HUMMING BREATH

This exercise will help restore calmness and balance to your system.

Sit on the floor in a comfortable position with your back straight. Close your eyes and breathe in deeply and hold for a few seconds. As you breathe out hum a 'mm' sound until you have expelled all the air. Direct the vibration of the 'mm' between your eyes. Repeat five times.

ALTERNATE NOSTRIL BREATH

It is thought that breathing through your nose can stimulate your endocrine system – important if you have PMS. It also helps the hypothalamus gland, which is responsible for nearly every function in your body, including mood and sleep. Whenever you feel tired or drained, try alternate nostril breathing, noticing how it refreshes you.

Sit comfortably and place your right hand on your face, resting the first two fingers over the bridge of your nose. You are going to use your thumb to block one nostril and your ring finger to block the other.

Breathe out of both nostrils. Then block your right nostril with your thumb and breathe in through your left nostril for a count of 5.

Now release your thumb and block your left nostril with your ring finger and breathe in through your right nostril for a count of 5.

Then breathe in through your right nostril, block it with your thumb, release your ring finger and breathe out through your left nostril. Carry on for about a minute.

EMOTIONAL WELL-BEING

Go for Goals

Setting goals is a great way to direct energy and enthusiasm back into your life. Today, spend a few moments thinking about your short-term and long-term goals. Your short-term goals should be manageable and very specific. They must be realistic and achievable within a time limit of around a year. Long-term goals have a wider time scale, for example three years. Their function is to give you something to aim towards. In business this is called the big picture or a mission statement focusing on the direction you want your life to go.

TIPS FOR GOAL-SETTING

For short-term goals, write down a list of the five things you would like to achieve over the next year. Stick to things which are manageable, like completing the 12-week plan, getting in touch with an old friend and so on.

If you just don't know what you want to do, think back to when you were a child. What were your dreams? Can you make some of them happen now?

For long-term goals, think about what you want to achieve over the next five years. Imagine you are nearly 90 years old. What have you done with your life? Or if you had five years left to live, how would you spend it? Is your life challenging enough? Write down your long-term goals and make sure that they are not too difficult to achieve. Travelling, having kids, working for a charity, changing jobs, moving house, learning a language or studying for a degree are all long-term goals you can consider.

Finally, don't be rigid about your goals. Your circumstances may change and you may need to change your goals to fit your lifestyle.

Day 4

NUTRITION

Enjoying a Smoothie
Try the delicious banana and strawberry smoothie recipe on page 214. (You'll find some more smoothie recipes in Appendix 4.) Strawberries are high in iron and are good for preventing anaemia; bananas are high in

potassium which is essential for all cell functions; calcium-enriched soya milk is not only full of calcium but also protein; linseeds contain essential fatty acids. All of these are great energy-boosters.

STRAWBERRY AND BANANA SMOOTHIE
10 fl oz/300 ml calcium-enriched soya milk
1 cup/230 g strawberries
1 banana
1 teaspoon linseeds
3 drops vanilla essence
Put everything in a blender and whiz for a few seconds – delicious!

EXERCISE

Go Rowing!
Do your 10-minute warm-up, your 20 minutes of vigorous exercise and your stretching. Then try this yoga exercise, designed to seal in and generate more energy.

ROWING EXERCISE

Sit on the floor with your legs out straight and imagine you are pulling the oars of a boat. Lean forward, arms outstretched, and breathe out. As you breathe in, pull on your imaginary oars as you lean back. Tighten your tummy and clench your buttocks, hold your breath and then move forward as you exhale. Repeat up to 10 times.

EMOTIONAL WELL-BEING

Give Yourself a Lift
Try to spend some time today – even if it's just 5 minutes – in surroundings and company that boost your self-esteem and energy. Take a walk in the park, phone a friend who makes you laugh – or, if that isn't possible, daydream for a few minutes about your ideal holiday. Why not

bring a bunch of flowers home with you today? It's a good way to delight your senses and raise your spirits.

Day 5

NUTRITION

Energy Menu
If you feel there is some way to go to balance your energy levels, here's a sample menu. Notice how the protein and fat balance the complex carbohydrates to give you more energy for longer and stop you getting those exhausting energy lows or food cravings that can play havoc with your blood sugar levels and make symptoms of PMS worse.

Breakfast with multivitamin: Scrambled eggs on whole meal toast, glass of calcium-enriched soya milk
Eggs provide a good source of protein and wholewheat toast is high in B vitamins needed for energy.
Snack: Rice cakes with almond butter, glass of calcium-enriched soya milk.
Almonds are a great source of protein, and in butter form are easily digested.
Almond butter is available from healthfood shops and some larger supermarkets.
Lunch: Vegetable and lentil soup with a salad and curd cheese sandwich.
Lentils, tomatoes and vegetables are high-energy foods packed with nutrients.
Curd cheese is low in fat and easily digested. The lentils and the bread are a good source of protein and fibre.
Snack: Banana and a handful of nuts and raisins
Both bananas and raisins are complex carbohydrates which help keep your energy levels high.
Dinner: Fish or tofu pie and spinach followed by baked apples
Combining the protein in fish with mashed potatoes will help keep your blood sugar stable.

EXERCISE

Upside-down Thinking

Do your 30-minute walk, your toning and your stretching – then try this inverted posture energy-boost. An inverted posture means that your head is lower than your heart, which encourages circulation to your upper body. In other words, your brain is supplied with fresh blood and oxygen to help wake you up.

> Lie on the floor with your legs resting on a chair for about a minute. You may hear a rushing to your ears as blood flows to your head. If it feels uncomfortable in any way, just come out of the position gently.

EMOTIONAL WELL-BEING

Tune In to the Music

Tune in to the healing power of music today. Many spiritual traditions use sound vibrations to calm the emotions, still the mind and restore inspiration. Think of the smooth reverential tones of Gregorian chants. Music can be very relaxing – or a rousing symphony may be just what you need to feel motivated, renewed and energized.

Ask yourself today 'What kind of music makes me feel better?' You may want to compile your own tape or CD that you can play as a daily mood-enhancer, or create a collection of tapes or CDs to match your needs: calming, energetic, romantic and so on.

Day 6

NUTRITION

A Detox Weekend

> Detoxing for a day or so every month has given me renewed confidence in
> my appearance, more energy to cope with the demands of my busy life
> and, for once in my life, the belief that I can change my eating habits and
> my life for the better. Detox starts with a change in diet but it is about
> healing not just the body but the mind and the soul. I feel lighter and
> happier afterwards. **Debby, 40**

Detoxing is a method used to help your body function more efficiently
and increase energy levels. The weekend detox regime we are going to
recommend is gentle and effective. If you don't feel ready for a gentle
detox yet or don't think you need it, no problem. You can always try it
later.

A good detox works with your kidneys, liver, skin and lymphatic system to
eliminate toxins in your body. The 2-day detox we are recommending will
enhance circulation, improve your immune system and clean your system
from the inside out.

Don't do this detox if you have had a stressful week, as there could be
side-effects that you may not be ready to cope with. These include spots,
bad breath and headaches – signs that toxins are being eliminated and
the programme is working – so make sure you are good to yourself and
take plenty of time for rest and relaxation during your detox. It's a good
idea to soak in a long hot bath at the end of each day with a few drops of
calming essential oil, like lavender, and make sure you get lots of sleep.

You may want to combine your detox with dry skin brushing, which will
help boost your lymphatic system and thereby speed up the elimination
of waste. Before you shower in the morning, spend a few minutes
brushing your body with a long-handled brush towards your heart. You

may also want to stimulate your skin and circulation by massaging with essential oils.

You should return to a normal diet on Monday. We are suggesting a weekend, but any two days when you don't have many commitments will be ideal. If your blood sugar levels are still all over the place, or if you are ill, you need to wait until your blood sugars are level or you feel well again.

You can eat as much organic fruit and vegetables as you like on your two-day detox. Drink as much water as you can, too.

Day 1
Breakfast with supplements: Fresh fruit (not bananas) with linseeds sprinkled on the top, cup of ginger tea to help boost circulation
Snack: Handful of sunflower seeds
Lunch: Artichoke and lemon salad
Snack: Organic diluted fresh-pressed apple juice
Dinner: Large plate of vegetables roasted in the oven with olive oil and some cooked brown rice sprinkled with seeds.

EXERCISE

Take a Deep Breath
Do your 30-minute walk today and your stretching. As you walk – hopefully in the fresh air to maximize your oxygen intake – don't forget to breathe properly. Most of us don't inflate our lungs fully, missing out on vital oxygen. Exhale completely, then slowly breathe in, allowing air to fill right to the bottom of your lungs so that your belly expands. Exhale again. Repeat for 10 minutes a day to give your energy levels a boost.

EMOTIONAL WELL-BEING

Discover Your Energy-sappers
Many things can cause fatigue, so if lack of energy is a real problem for you, have a think about the following useful tips:

Are you sleeping well? If not, you might want to read our tips about getting a good night's sleep on pages 173–6.

Are you drinking tea and coffee during the day? Read our tips on cutting down on caffeine on page 56.

Are you passionate about something? When you are focused and motivated you feel alert and energized. Recently this truth has been corroborated by psychologist Mihalyi Csikszentmihalyi at the University of Chicago. He has written a groundbreaking book called *Flow: The Psychology of Optimal Living*. Flow is the experience of true enjoyment and absorption in a task. What are these for you? Gardening, dancing, working on a car, playing an instrument, running, playing with your kids, singing in a choir, teaching, painting, helping someone? See if you can identify your 'flow' experiences, and then bring them into your daily or weekly routine.

What about your iron levels? Reread information from the beginning of this week.

Are you stressed? Follow our advice on pages 88–91 for managing stress.

Are you eating nutritious meals and snacks throughout the day? Remember, five or six meals and snacks total.

Are you active enough? If you feel too tired, exercise may be just want you need to feel invigorated.

Is there another cause? If fatigue persists you may have a food intolerance (see page 185) or there could be another cause such as thyroid problems, candida or diabetes. We'll discuss these possibilities later in the plan. You may find it helpful to turn to our A-Z of PMS symptoms to check out the advice there and to explore various remedies for fatigue.

Day 7

NUTRITION

Detox Day 2
Breakfast with supplements: Fresh fruit with linseeds, cup of ginger tea
Snack: Lemon with fruit juice, olive oil and garlic (a detoxifying lemon drink)
Lunch: Vegetable soup with onions, carrots and celery; three-bean salad
Snack: Glass of organic, diluted apple juice
Dinner: Large plate of steamed vegetables with cooked brown rice sprinkled with almonds or cashews

EXERCISE

No walk or toning today, but do your stretching routine or your yoga poses. Yoga and stretching can help realign your body, allowing vital energy to flow freely. And after your yoga session, or whenever you feel like it, make time to soak for at least 15 minutes in a warm bath with aromatherapy oils.

EMOTIONAL WELL-BEING

Plan for Happiness
Learning to manage your time is the secret to creating a lifestyle that truly nurtures and supports you.

Alan Lakein's classic book, *How to Get Control of Your Time and Your Life,* shows that successful time-management begins with making a list of what is most important in your life. After listing your priorities, you set your goals by assigning an A to those items that have a high value, a B to those of medium value and a C to those with the lowest value. Finally you block out periods of time each day to work on those high-priority A goals.

You may at this point in the plan want to create your own healthy self-care daily activity schedule with hours marked from the time you get up to the time you go to bed. You'll find an example at the end of the book you might want to photocopy. This schedule is for you to write down those priority self-care activities that have become part of your daily routine and that you want to ensure you make regular time for.

VITALITY BOOSTER

Let There Be Light!
Have you ever noticed how great you feel when it is a beautiful sunny day? You feel eager to go out and live. Then think about how you feel when you wake up in wintertime – it's dark and cold and raining. Isn't it depressing to get out of bed?

Many women find that their symptoms of PMS get more severe when the days are darker or shorter, as the lack of warmth and light makes things worse. But why should PMS be connected to light? We've already looked at melatonin, which shifts your body into a lower gear and makes you feel sleepy. When you are exposed to bright light your body starts to produce serotonin, which wakes you up and makes you feel more alert, energetic and happy. Without enough serotonin you can end up feeling depressed and irritable, with food cravings, and you have problems sleeping. Sounds a bit like PMS, doesn't it? In fact, research has shown that serotonin/melatonin levels actually drop in order for ovulation to occur.

It's clear that too little serotonin and melatonin, as well as too little light, can play a part in PMS or make it worse. Here's a checklist of the symptoms caused by both:

- a change of appetite
- difficulty sleeping
- low self-esteem
- reduced energy
- weight gain
- difficulty concentrating
- fatigue

So light up your life. This is especially important if your PMS tends to get worse in the winter or if you suffer from depression. By boosting your serotonin and melatonin levels, your mood is lighter and you have more energy.

To increase your serotonin production, make sure you are exposed to either full-spectrum light from the sun or a bright white light. The incandescent lights you may have in your lamps just aren't the same. Walk outdoors for about 10 minutes each day – preferably in the morning. Don't wear sunglasses so your eyes will be exposed to the (indirect) light rays.

If you think you need something more, you might want to consider getting a special light box that can provide fluorescent full-spectrum light, or a bright white light that contains no UV wavelengths (UV can cause skin cancer). There are also new systems that use cool-white and bi-axial lamps. The light is measured in units called *lux*, and a typical light box provides 10,000 lux. Daylight is around 5,000 lux and it takes around 2,500 lux to have a therapeutic effect on your internal clock. You can do light therapy yourself as long as you follow the instructions with your box to the letter and don't overdo it – but it is always best to check with your doctor first for advice.

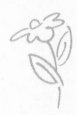

Week 9

Day 1

NUTRITION

Think Organic
This week as you plan and buy and eat your healthy menu (don't forget
that multivitamin and -mineral and calcium and magnesium supplement
every day), we'd like you to think about organic food.

Why is organic food good if you have PMS? Because conventionally-grown
foods contain xenoestrogens, which are oestrogen-like chemicals present
in pesticides and plastics. They are stored in body fat and can rob food of
its energy potential and upset your hormonal balance. In wildlife the
dramatic effects of xenoestrogens are seen in fish growing both male and
female sex organs. In our environment[1] we are seeing girls enter puberty
earlier and earlier, and this has been linked to a diet too high in synthetic
hormones. Xenoestrogens may be at the root of many female hormone
problems, including PMS.

Since in Britain and the US most vegetables and fruits are sprayed before they reach the supermarket shelves, buy as much organic food as you can. Organic foods are produced without using chemicals, pesticides or fertilizers, all of which have been linked to conditions such as cancer, infertility and PMS. Organic farm animals are reared humanely and not pumped full of growth hormones and antibiotics, and they have good access to food, water and the outdoors.

To avoid xenoestrogens from plastics leaching into your food, buy drinks in glass bottles, don't heat food in the microwave if it's in plastic packaging, and avoid PVC where you can. Filter your water.

EXERCISE

Ready to Revamp?
Is your exercise routine still challenging you or have you hit a plateau? Many people need an exercise pick-me-up around two months into their programme.

For starters, begin to keep an exercise diary. People who keep fitness diaries tend to make faster progress with their exercise routine and can see the progress they're making. Starting today, after every workout add a fitness section into your emotions diary. Include the exercises completed and how you felt during the workout. Gauge your results by comparing today's performance against next week's. Are you doing too much of the same thing? Is it too easy for you? That means you are getting into better shape whether you realize it or not. Remember how far you have come and how much better you feel than before you started exercising. Congratulate yourself on what you have done so far, then think of ways to move on.

EMOTIONAL WELL-BEING

Treat Yourself – You're Nearly There!
This week we are going to remind you about lots of tips to feel happy and healthy every day. At this crucial stage in the 12-week plan, you are so

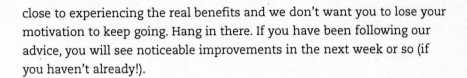

close to experiencing the real benefits and we don't want you to lose your motivation to keep going. Hang in there. If you have been following our advice, you will see noticeable improvements in the next week or so (if you haven't already!).

Be good to yourself. Take time out for a leisurely meal out or a self-pampering night in. Guilt depresses your immune system, so allow yourself relaxation and enjoyment. You deserve it.

Stand tall. Good posture will help you look and feel better. Imagine an invisible thread lifting you from the top of your head. Alexander Technique expert Glynn Macdonald recommends this exercise: 'When standing, loosen your neck by moving your head gently up and then down to your chest. Let your knees stay soft, not locked. Try not to hold your breath or let your weight sink into your hips.'

Express yourself. Nourish your soul and relieve your mind by getting creative today. Do some painting, singing or dancing. Write in your mood diary. Explore your emotions through movement – a dance class, a tai chi class, or just running in the park.

Day 2

NUTRITION

Turn Shop Detective

If you get a chance today or sometime this week, why not pop round to your nearest supermarket and check out their organic range – they are bound to have one. You could also pay a visit to your local healthfood shop. If you need to top up on fruits, vegetables and dairy produce, why not try the organic alternatives?

EXERCISE

Overcoming a Block

If you feel stuck with your exercise routine, it may be time to reassess your goals. Your long-term goals need to be beyond your current abilities, but not so far off that you lose motivation. Are your long-term fitness goals realistic?

If you have longer-term goals, break them down into smaller bite-sized pieces. If you want to run a marathon, start with gently jogging for 10 minutes. When you can do that comfortably, buy yourself a small present, such as a book, a CD or a bunch of flowers as a way of congratulating yourself. Then set a new goal of running twice that time. You'll make the best progress when you work towards a series of short-term goals and reward yourself regularly.

Grab your fitness diary and, after your workout today, write down some short-term goals. A weight loss of 2 kilos, not 10, mastering two yoga postures, not all of them, lifting light weights, not heavy ones, doing 20 minutes of vigorous exercise 2 times a week, not 5, and so on. And when you successfully achieve these small goals, don't forget to reward yourself before you sit down to set new small goals.

EMOTIONAL WELL-BEING

Clear Your Head

A clear head and good concentration help you deal with challenges and boost your feelings of well-being.

- Use coloured objects to inspire clear thinking. In Feng Shui, yellow stimulates the mind and red helps you to focus.
- Don't forget to stock up on your B vitamins, found in wholegrains or taken as a supplement. B vitamins are vital for mental health.
- Peppermint essential oil can also boost mental performance. Put a few drops on a tissue and sniff a couple of times for 5 minutes.

Day 3

NUTRITION

The Organic Health Boost

Organic food certainly looks and tastes better than conventional food, but is it really better for your health?

The answer is *yes*. Studies have shown that chemicals that cause cancer and pesticides and can interfere with hormonal balance have been found in our food supplies and our water. There is also certain evidence that organic food is higher in certain nutrients, including potassium and vitamin C.

If you just can't afford organic foods, take preventative measures. Wash and peel all fruit and vegetables. Stick with fresh, whole foods as much as you can instead of processed and refined versions, and perhaps try and have just one organic food choice a week.

EXERCISE

Change Your Routine

Variety is the spice of life, so here are some suggestions to revamp your routine.

- Buy a skipping rope. You are more likely to exercise if you have fun at the same time.
- Go swimming instead of your walk or run: It doesn't stress your muscles and joints in the same way.
- Cross-training: In cross-training you engage in two or more types of exercise, either in one workout or one week. Professional athletes cross-train all the time so they don't do the same exercises every day.

Sample Cross-training Programme

Monday: 30-min brisk walk, stretch, upper-body toning
Tuesday: 10-min walk, 20-min light jog, stretch, lower-body weight-training

Wednesday: Swimming and yoga
Thursday: Cycling or playing sport, stretching
Friday: 30-min brisk walk, upper- and lower-body toning
Saturday: 30-min jog, stretching
Sunday: Leisurely stroll

EMOTIONAL WELL-BEING

Time for Pleasure

Take time today to seek fun and pleasure. Rent a funny video or do something fun like ice-skating with a friend or sharing a joke over coffee.

Sex is a great mood-enhancer – and great exercise.

Laughter helps lower levels of the stress hormone cortisol. And if all else fails, treat yourself to some chocolate to trigger the release of some feel-good endorphins.

Day 4

NUTRITION

Finding Local Suppliers

Hopefully you're convinced to include more organic food in your diet. But where can you buy it? We've already mentioned your local supermarket – they will have an organic range and you can get everything under one roof. Box schemes and farmer's markets are other good ways to buy organic cheaply. The method also supports the local community and ensures that organic produce isn't imported. For details of both, see our Resources chapter.

Your local healthfood shop should stock everything from cereals to baby foods, organic cakes and sweets, so this is another good place to try. You may also find that lots of companies on the Internet can have anything from food and wine to skincare products and nappies delivered to your door.

EXERCISE

Interval Time

Another way to add variety to your exercise routine is interval training, which is a method of varying the intensity of your workout. Short bursts of vigorous activity are alternated with less intense exercise. You can interval train with any aerobic exercise. For example, you go all-out for one minute and then return to your normal pace. Then 5 minutes later you go all-out again and return to your normal pace again.

Do interval training once or twice a week and you'll move out of your plateau.

When you start with interval training, your interval-to-rest ratio should be 1 to 3, so if you exercise intensely for 1 minute you should recover for 3 minutes.

Try this interval workout in your routine. Do it today and again on Day 6:

- Warm up with a brisk walk for 20 minutes.
- Run as fast as you can for 20 seconds.
- Slow down and walk for 1 minute.
- Repeat this interval-and-recovery programme six more times.
- Stretch to cool down.

EMOTIONAL WELL-BEING

Stress Check

Take a walk in the park or find a quiet place to do your breathing exercises today. If you haven't already, switch from tea and coffee to herbal teas. And put things into perspective. Professor Stephen Palmer, Director of the Centre for Stress-management, advises 'Ask yourself, how serious will it be if this task is not done?'

Day 5

NUTRITION

A Glass of Wine
When you go shopping this week, why not buy and sample a bottle of
organic wine? Conventional wines have been found to contain hundreds
of chemicals, but organic wines use cover-crops to attract wildlife to eat
the insects that can destroy crops. And most are suitable for vegetarians.

EXERCISE

More Choice!
Another way to inject variety and challenge into your exercise routine is
to apply the hard/easy principle to your exercise routine. Exercise
intensely two or three times a week and less intensely on other days. So
you have two or three tougher workouts – such as jogging or cycling –
which make your muscles ache a little, and easier recovery days with a
walk or a swim when you don't push yourself. This is based on the theory
that your muscle groups need 48 hours to recover from exercise.

EMOTIONAL WELL-BEING

Rejuvenate!
Do you sometimes feel much older than you are, especially when PMS is
really bad? Here are some simple tips to help you feel physically and
mentally younger.

- Give your complexion a glow with a massage. Wash your hands and
  then use them both to sweep the skin upwards from your neck to
  forehead and then out to the sides. Gently pinch your face from
  cheekbones to jawline. Stroke up from your brows to your hairline,
  then smooth your hands over your entire face. For more ideas read
  Natural Facelifts by Juliette Kando.
- Focus on your child within. Children take every moment as it comes
  and see the fun in everything. How could you enjoy this moment?

- Eat more broccoli and dark fruits such as black grapes which are rich in anti-ageing antioxidants like vitamin C.
- Ensure your diet is sufficient in iron. Good sources include lentils and soya beans.
- Get out and meet people. Having fun with friends at the end of the day is an antidote to unpleasant experiences during the day.
- Don't forget your daily exercise. If you can't manage the full 30 minutes, a few bursts of gentle exercise spread throughout the day are almost as effective as one long burst.

Day 6

NUTRITION

Go Chemical-free
- Avoid, as much as you can, food and drink in plastic containers. Don't wrap or heat food in plastic. Why? Because xenoestrogens found in plastic are fat-loving and tend to migrate towards food with a high-fat content. If you do buy food wrapped in plastic, remove it as soon as you can.
- Watch your intake of saturated fat. Xenoestrogens live in fat stores and you don't want to provide a home for them.
- Increase your intake of fibre (see pages 118–19) to prevent the absorption of unwanted chemicals into your bloodstream.
- Eat more cruciferous vegetables like broccoli, Brussels sprouts, cauliflower and cabbage.
- Eat phytoestrogens. You may want to re-read page 22 here. Foods such as soya, lentils and chickpeas can reduce the toxic form of oestrogen in your body.
- Avoid products that have been genetically modified (GM). Stick to organic produce and other foods that have not been tampered with.
- Use organic toiletries and cosmetics. Up to 60 per cent of what you put on your skin makes its way into your bloodstream. (That's why patches are used to deliver nicotine or HRT.)
- Buy natural cleaning products for your home to cut down on the number of potentially toxic substances in your environment.

- Buy organic clothes. They are free from chemicals, which can irritate your skin.

EXERCISE

Spark Up with a Circuit

Circuit-training is another way to breathe new life into your exercise routine. The circuit-training format uses a group of exercises that are completed in sequence, one right after another. Each exercise is performed for a specified number of repetitions or time period before you move on to the next exercise. There are little or no rest intervals between exercises, but there are short periods of rest between each completed circuit.

Depending on your fitness levels you may perform between two and six circuits.

Here's a sample circuit. Look over the list and make sure you have enough room to do all the exercises. Repeat each exercise for 45 seconds, with 15 seconds in between to transition to the next. Don't count how many exercises you do, just focus on getting through those 45 seconds. Remember that as you get fitter you can always adjust your timing.

Jog on the spot for 5 minutes to warm up. Follow this with stretching. For details on how to do the various toning exercises see page 163.
Squats (45 seconds); 15-second transition
Sit-ups (45 seconds); 15-second transition
Push-ups (45 seconds); 15-second transition
Jumping jacks or skipping (45 seconds); 15-second transition
Lunges (45 seconds); 15-second transition
Obliques (45 seconds); 30-second transition.
Repeat entire circuit sequence two to four times.

EMOTIONAL WELL-BEING

Mood Check

Take a moment today to check on your mood. How do you feel about your achievements so far? If you feel good, that's great. If you don't feel good or feel that you haven't achieved as much as you'd like, don't beat yourself up. Remember the power is always in the present moment. Every moment is a fresh beginning. You can take steps today, right now, to get yourself back on track.

Day 7

NUTRITION

Try organic free-range eggs. Free-range is certainly kinder on the hens. If you are on a limited budget and are unsure of what to prioritize when you go shopping for organic produce, buy fruit and vegetables first then organic grains such as brown rice or wholemeal bread. This will make a huge difference. Grains are very small and can absorb a lot of toxins, and fruit and veg are the foundation stones of your diet.

Finally, remember that organic produce like carrots and potatoes, unlike conventional produce, does not have to be peeled. Most of the nutrients in fruits and vegetables are just under the skin, so all you need to do is wash them and prepare as normal.

EXERCISE

Don't Overdo It!

This week we have looked at ways you can add variety to your exercise routine to keep your motivation going and see your fitness levels constantly improve. But beware of overexercising, which can make you feel tired, irritable and more vulnerable to infection. Train for no more than six or seven hours a week, and make sure you always have one day when you take it easy.

How do you know if you have been overdoing it? Here are some signs to watch out for:

- exercise leaves you feeling exhausted not energized
- your fitness isn't improving
- you aren't as coordinated as usual
- you get regular aches and pains
- your stomach hurts and you get ill often
- you lose your appetite
- you feel depressed and apathetic
- your self-esteem is low.

If you notice any of the above, it is time to lighten the load or take a break for a short while. As with everything in the plan, moderation is key.

EMOTIONAL WELL-BEING

Tiny Tips – Big Results!

As today is probably your rest day, here are some quick and easy ways to help balance mind, body and spirit.

- Use colour therapy: Wear red for energy, orange for happiness, yellow for concentration and blue for relaxation. Paint a room: Opt for yellow and orange in social rooms and green or blue to aid a more restful environment.
- Use Bach Flower Remedies to ease your emotions. Try Rock Water if you demand too much of yourself, Pine if you tend to take other people's guilt on board too much.
- Put a clear crystal quartz in your bathroom to balance your emotions.
- Take some 'me' time. Plan some pampering time and indulge in a long soak in your bath. Add a few drops of lavender oil to a warm bath and focus on relaxing every muscle from your toes to your forehead.
- Adopt a mantra to focus on when you find yourself feeling anxious. Close your eyes and repeat a word or phrase to yourself to distract your mind from the stress. For example 'I am relaxed,' 'I feel good.'

VITALITY BOOSTER

The Healing Power of Love and Friendship

'If you feel depressed or lonely, you're three to five times more likely to pick up illnesses than people who have a sense of love and connection with someone else,' says Dr Dean Ornish, author of *Love and Survival: How good relationships can bring you health and well-being.*

Our health depends on the healing power of love, intimacy and relationships. If you have PMS, the healing power of love may be just what you need to ease symptoms and get your life back on track. Good relationships give you a sense of belonging and attachment. If you are not in a relationship you can get the same effect from spending time with close friends or family, or even your pet.

- Loving thoughts and acts can make you feel better about yourself and boost your well-being. If you feel ill or down, try to be with someone who cares about you, or be extra caring towards yourself. When you get into a loving state of mind, the nervous system sends healthy, positive messages to your brain and immune system.
- Regular sex isn't just good exercise – research shows that sex helps to relieve insomnia and stress because it stimulates the release of feel-good endorphins. Sexual arousal also produces powerful hormones which encourages strong bonds with your partner.
- Perfect relationships don't exist, so enjoy the value of real relationships. For relationships to become really strong and intimate, the two of you need to learn to value each other's differences and get through the tough times as well.
- Being touched boosts your well-being and immunity. Studies of HIV patients have shown that those who remain in close relationships stay healthier for longer. Babies who are hugged and held develop a lot earlier and faster than those who are not. So get hugging, holding hands, a kiss or a massage today.
- Heal your heart by sharing your feelings more. Write in your mood journal, talk to people you trust or join a support group.

- Learn how to forgive. If you are carrying a grudge, make a point to drop it. Forgiving others does not excuse their behaviour but it frees you from the negative effects of anger on yourself.
- Develop your spiritual life. Believing in a power greater than yourself allows you to feel part of and loved by a larger community.
- Prayer and meditation can give you a higher level of interconnection with others. Dr Ornish defines love 'as anything that takes you out of the experience of being separate'. And a powerful way to do that is to commune with God or whatever name you give to that experience.
- Make a commitment. Commitment to another gives you a safe zone in which you can be vulnerable, and vulnerability makes greater intimacy possible.

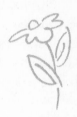

Week 10

Day 1

NUTRITION

In Week 1 of the plan, we explained that even if you eat a healthy diet you still need to take supplements to help fight PMS. This is because – and surveys[1] back this up – the vast majority of us will not get the nutrients we need from the food we eat.

In addition to your daily multivitamin and -mineral and your additional calcium and magnesium supplement, this week we will also look at the healing power of herbal supplements you might like to try.

Warning: If you are thinking about starting a family, avoid any kind of herbal treatment unless you have consulted and are under the supervision of a qualified specialist. And because some supplements can cause side-effects it is always best to read labels carefully. Check the Resources chapter for websites with further information.

Camomile (Matricaria chamomile)

We've mentioned camomile tea for its relaxing qualities, but the herb also has natural anti-inflammatory, antibacterial and antifungal ingredients. Camomile has been used for centuries to treat insomnia, aches and pains and anxiety. If you are not allergic to members of the aster or daisy family, try a cup of camomile tea (made from one tablespoon of camomile flower steeped in boiling water) three times a day, or take 10 to 20 drops of extract mixed with water two to three times a day.

Dandelion (Taraxacum officinale)

Loaded with betacarotene, vitamin C, iron, calcium, potassium and other minerals, the dandelion is an excellent diuretic that helps your body shed the excess water that contributes to PMS bloating, and helps to stabilize blood sugar levels. Dandelion stimulates and supports liver function, which is important for the breakdown of toxins and old hormones. Constipation, headaches and acne can be eased with this herb. Almost the whole plant – flowers, leaves and root – can be used for herbal treatments. Juice can be extracted from the plant; the leaves can be eaten; tea can be made from the roots or leaves. You can also get tinctures and extracts from healthfood shops.

Nettle

You may not want to have anything to do with nettles, but this versatile herb has been used for centuries. Herbalists consider the nettle a great all-round tonic for women with PMS, especially for its diuretic properties and its high nutrient content. You can take nettles as a tincture, juice or tea, but you can also eat freshly cooked nettle greens (nettles are available at some healthfood shops).

Chasteberry (Vitex agnus-castus)

Chasteberry tree extract helps to balance your hormones by binding to dopamine receptors in the pituitary gland. This in turn reduces your production of prolactin. Because prolactin and progesterone tend to balance each other, reducing prolactin boosts your progesterone, and this can ease PMS. Three large studies[2] on a total of 4,500 women on the effect of chasteberry extract on PMS showed that at a daily dosage of 40 drops of liquid extract (35 mg of plant extract), nearly one-third of the women found relief and more than half saw marked improvement.

Warning: If you are taking the Pill, avoid chasteberry as its effect on prolactin could end up decreasing the Pill's effectiveness.

Black Cohosh (Cimifuga racemosa)

Black Cohosh has oestrogen-like actions that appear to rebalance female hormones. Because it can occupy oestrogen-receptor sites it has the ability to lower high oestrogen levels and reduce the effects of oestrogen dominance. In women with low oestrogen levels, Black Cohosh can supply a mild oestrogenic boost. As well as balancing hormones it also has a calming effect on the nervous system and can be helpful with PMS anxiety, stress and depression. It also is a mild painkiller and is useful for PMS headaches.

Warning: It is better to avoid this herb if you get heavy periods.

Dong Quai (Angelica sinensis)

This Chinese herb, known as the female ginseng, has a long history. It can be helpful with PMS because studies[3] show that it promotes hormonal balance and can regulate sugar levels. It appears to have phytoestrogen effects which are helpful when the problem is too much or too little oestrogen. And because Dong Quai also has muscle-relaxing qualities it is particularly suggested for women who get premenstrual pains and cramps.

EXERCISE

Day Off!

If you tried the suggestions we recommended last week to spice up your fitness routine, you have done a lot of physical exercise – so give yourself a day off from exercise today.

EMOTIONAL WELL-BEING

Boosting Your Self-esteem

Good self-esteem isn't something you are born with but something you need to learn in life, and this week we are going to give you some confidence-boosting strategies that you can use any time. We've already mentioned affirmations, like:

> *I am a healthy woman.*
> *I am fun to be around.*
> *I am in charge of my life.*
> *I am a success.*

– now here's a little exercise we'd like you to try today.

Just for fun, see how many positive affirmations you can write down about yourself in 5 minutes. Then, whenever you feel low, take out your list and study it. Better still, stick your list somewhere you can see it often.

Day 2

NUTRITION

Continuing our herbal supplement theme, here are some more herbs commonly used to treat PMS which you might like to think about when you next browse at your local healthfood shop or chemist.

False Unicorn Root

This herb is known to be help restore hormonal balance and function. It exerts a mild oestrogen-like effect, boosting low levels or lowering high ones. False unicorn root is also believed to ease headaches and treat delayed periods.

Milk Thistle (Silybum marianum)

If you have PMS, support for the liver is important, since this detoxifying organ plays a big part in the breakdown and excretion of unwanted oestrogen. The liver also detoxifies harmful substances such as alcohol, nicotine and other toxins.

Motherwort (Lenourus cardiaca)
Way back in the 17th century motherwort was highly regarded as a tonic
for menstrual pains and labour pains. Motherwort is recommended by
herbalists today for delayed menstruation, water-retention, nervous
tension and to generally ease symptoms of PMS.

EXERCISE

Start-up Time
After your two-day break from exercise you should be bursting with
energy and raring to go. Do your 30-minute brisk walk, your stretching
and your toning today, then spend some time thinking about how far you
have come in the last 10 weeks. Can you do more than you could back in
Week 1? Is your 30-minute walk getting easier? Do you feel fitter? If you
can see definite progress, well done. If you can't, later this week we'll give
you some tips to help you improve. Tomorrow we'll do a fitness test, so
make sure you get a good night's sleep tonight.

EMOTIONAL WELL-BEING

Feeling Confident
Today, play 'let's pretend'. Appear calm today even if you don't feel it.
Before you enter a room, collect yourself, stand tall and walk purposefully.
Maintain eye contact with the people you meet and speak in a warm,
expressive tone. A smile not only makes you look confident, it also helps
relax you so that you actually feel more confident.

Wear confident colours. Wear orange close to your face (say, in a scarf) on
big occasions. Light pink and red are also good when you want to give a
confident impression. Blue and turquoise aid communication, so they are
ideal colours to wear to work.

Day 3

NUTRITION

Sound Familiar?
If herbal supplements sound daunting and unfamiliar try some well-known herbal remedies, like the camomile, nettle or dandelion listed earlier.

EXERCISE

Test Your Fitness
Do your 10-minute warm-up and your stretching, then grab a tape measure. While standing, exhale normally (don't suck your stomach in) and measure your waist at the belly button. Now measure your hips at their widest part – usually around your backside. Now divide your waist measurement by your hip measurement to get your waist-to-hip ratio. If your ratio is less than 0.80 you are in the healthy range. If you are between 0.80 and 0.85 you are borderline. Over 0.85 is unhealthy.

The waist-to-hip ratio is a good indicator of health and fitness, because where you store your fat is an important health factor. People who are heavier in the middle are more at risk of health problems – such as diabetes and heart disease – even compared to people who are equally fat but whose fat is more evenly distributed. Just make a note of your ratio now and move on to your next test – muscle strength.

Drop down on your hands and knees and do as many push-ups as you can. Then do the same for your crunches. Have a think back to Week 1. Do you think you have improved? If you have, well done. If you haven't, don't worry, we'll give you some advice tomorrow. Time for your next test.

Stand up straight with your feet shoulder-width apart. Bend at the waist reaching towards the floor, but don't bend your knees. Notice how far you can reach. Once again, think back to Week 1. Have you improved?

Finally, it's time for your aerobics test. Make sure you warm up and then run, walk or jog at a steady pace for 3.3 km or 1.5 miles on a flat surface. (Six laps around a typical quarter-mile/half-kilometre running track.) Time how long it takes you. If you don't feel you can go that far yet, pace yourself. However long it takes you, you should feel tired at the end, but not weak. How long did it take you? If you did it under 13 minutes, your fitness level is superior. If you did it under 16½ minutes, you are doing OK. If you took over 17 minutes there is still some way to go to improve your fitness.

Don't worry. Whatever your level of fitness, there is plenty of time to improve.

EMOTIONAL WELL-BEING

Take Up the Challenge
Today when you face a difficult situation, try to think of it as a challenge and not a problem. You are a creative and resourceful person and you can rise above whatever life challenges you with.

The Chinese symbol for crisis is also the symbol for opportunity. What an interesting way to think about PMS! Instead of being a problem it becomes a challenge to your inventiveness. Rising to the challenge of PMS has given you an opportunity to improve your health in all areas of your life. The problem of PMS becomes an opportunity for you to grow, develop and take control of your health and your life.

Day 4

NUTRITION
Both of these herbs are noted for their calming, soothing effect – and don't we all need that from time to time?

St John's Wort
St John's Wort has been used as a medicinal herb since Greek and Roman times, but only recently has it been rediscovered as a mood-enhancer for

those suffering from anxiety, mild depression and PMS-related symptoms. Researchers believe that St John's Wort can work as an anti-depressant without the side-effects of conventional medications. It helps make the feel-good chemicals – such as serotonin – more available. Although some women say they feel better in a matter of days, in general it takes about two to three months before the full benefits can be experienced.

Do not use alcohol or take any anti-depressant drug or the contraceptive pill if you use this herb.

Valerian

Calming Valerian is often recommended for PMS anxiety, stress and tension, and for the depression caused by stress or nervous tension. Valerian is well known as a sleep aid, and studies show that it can increase sleep quality because it shortens the amount of time it takes for you to fall asleep.

EXERCISE

More Fitness Testing

Do your 30-minute aerobic session, your toning and your stretching today, then think about the test you did yesterday. What did you learn?

If your waist-to-hip ratio was healthy, keep it up. If it was borderline or unhealthy, watch your portion size and make sure you do at least two to three 20-minute sessions of vigorous aerobic activity a week. You could also extend two of your daily workout times from 30 minutes of aerobic activity to 40 minutes, or sign up for an additional hour-long aerobics class that meets once a week. It might also be a good idea to step up your toning sessions from two to three or even four times a week. Crunches can certainly help you tone the mid-section, but you can't lose weight from one area only.

If you think your muscle strength has improved from Week 1, then you are heading in the right direction. If you haven't made much progress, add a few extra push-ups to your morning routine, get some light weights and work out while you watch your favourite soap. The same applies to your crunches and other toning work.

How was your stretching? If you are more flexible, well done. If not, try adding a few gentle stretches to your bedtime routine. It feels good and will help you sleep better.

Finally, how are you doing with your aerobic fitness? If you are still having problems, just stick at it. At your own pace keep gently increasing the time and intensity of your aerobic workout and make sure that you exercise aerobically every day.

EMOTIONAL WELL-BEING

Stay Away from Grumpy People

Do you know someone who is always complaining? Do you enjoy spending time with them? We bet you don't. If there is someone in your life who makes you feel depressed, stay away. This person is determined that they (and you) will never have a good day. They are victims of life and want to stay that way – but you don't.

Day 5

NUTRITION

Cookbooks

Have a look through your recipe books, or ones in the bookshop or library, and see if there are any new ones you'd like to try. Make a list of any ingredients and plan them in for Saturday.

EXERCISE

Each to Her Own

Enjoy your exercise session today and use the information from yesterday to style your routine to your particular needs. Try to keep your fitness goals realistic and remember that everyone is different and responds at their own rate to a new routine.

EMOTIONAL WELL-BEING

Imagination
Try this affirmation – an active day-dream to boost your motivation and happiness.

Find 5 minutes of quiet time in a place you won't be disturbed. Close your eyes and relax. Follow your breathing until you feel deeply relaxed, then see yourself happy and healthy, living a PMS-free life. You look so confident and relaxed; you feel positive about your day. See people treating you with the respect that you deserve. Make the vision as real as you can: see and hear the whole thing in glorious Technicolor, create the sound effects, feel the reality of your health, happiness and success.

When you are ready, let your thoughts return, open your eyes and come back to the room.

Days 6 and 7

NUTRITION

Herbal Remedy Review
All this week we have focused on herbal supplements you can take in addition to your multi-vitamin and -mineral. You may at this point want to read our A - Z of Symptoms. In addition to the advice and information given there about the most common PMS symptoms and natural ways to treat them, you'll find more recommended herbal remedies.

EXERCISE

Be Your Own Personal Fitness Trainer!
This weekend find a spare moment to sit down and think about your
fitness goals for the month ahead. Plan your fitness routine for a week
and then repeat that four times. Remember, however fit you are you will
still need to do some aerobic exercise five or six days a week, toning work
three or four times a week, and stretching every day. Don't forget to add
lots of variety to your routine.

EMOTIONAL WELL-BEING

Give Yourself a Treat!
Do something just for you today. Go to that class you want to, go to the
hairdressers, go for a swim, have an aromatherapy massage, stay in bed
all day, get a baby-sitter and go out to the cinema, read a book (or start
writing one), have a manicure or a pedicure. Anything you like. What
would you love to do but never seem to have the time for? Make the time
for it today and really enjoy it – you deserve it.

VITALITY BOOSTER

Alternative Therapies for PMS
Natural therapies aren't essential, but we thought you should have a fuller
picture of the options out there because some women have reported real
benefits. Alternative therapies are those not typically prescribed by medical
doctors, but any treatment you try has the potential to be dangerous if
used improperly – so here's a guide for evaluating alternative treatments:

- Beware of quick-fix treatments that offer to cure PMS.
- Avoid any treatment with an outrageous price tag.
- Think about who is selling you the treatment. Is it a doctor or natural
  health professional, or someone out to make a quick buck?

We've discussed light therapy, herbal supplements, massage and yoga.
Here are some other approaches to investigate to see if they benefit you.

ACUPUNCTURE

Acupuncture is part of the Chinese practice of medicine that involves using fine needles to regulate the flow of energy (called *chi*) in the body, stimulate the body's own healing responses and remove blockages of energy flow. The application of heat and massage may also be part of the process. Many women with PMS find it is helpful for relieving symptoms and boosting energy.

ACUPRESSURE

Instead of using needles to change the energy flow, the practitioner applies pressure to various body parts. Shiatsu is another practice that involves the application of pressure to energy pathways.

AROMATHERAPY

Aromatherapy oils are essential oils extracted from aromatic plants. Each essential oil works through your sense of smell and by being absorbed by the skin and lungs into your bloodstream, where it has a healing effect on organs, glands and tissues. With the exception of lavender and tea tree, essential oils should be blended with a carrier oil, such as almond oil, or diluted in water before coming into contact with your skin. Drops of essential oil can also be used directly in your bath or used as massage oil. (Some oils are not appropriate during pregnancy: Check with a qualified practitioner before using any oil if you think you may be pregnant.)

Pine, Rosemary, Sweet Fennel	Can relieve fear and anxiety
Clary Sage	Lifts mood
Fennel	Good for water-retention
Jasmine	Can ease tension and anxiety
Geranium	Has a cooling effect and can help with anxiety
Rosemary	Can help prevent fluid-retention
Bergamot and Camomile	Effective in reducing irritability and depression
Lavender	Helps to encourage a good night's sleep

HOMEOPATHY

Homeopathy is based on the concept of 'like cures like' in the same way that vaccinations do. If you are interested in homeopathy don't try and treat yourself, but visit a qualified practitioner.

Homeopathic remedies often prescribed for PMS:

Nux Vomica	For irritability and food cravings
Natrum Mur	For fluid-retention
Pulsatilla	For feeling tearful
Sepia	For irritability and depression

PSYCHOTHERAPY

For women with PMS, studies[4] show that cognitive therapy is a good way to address the condition's psychological effects, especially feelings of helplessness. The effects seem to last for several months after the sessions have finished. Cognitive behavioural therapy (CBT) is based on the belief that there is a direct relationship between the way we think, feel and behave. You are taught how to replace negative thought patterns with more positive, rational ones which in turn will help you regain control over your life.

REFLEXOLOGY

Points on your hands and feet are thought to correspond to various organs and systems in your body, and pressing on them is thought to correct imbalances in your body. Reflexology has been shown to help women with PMS. In one study[5] pressure in the correct places was applied to women in one group and in the incorrect places for women in another. The women who had the real reflexology showed a significant improvement in symptoms.

THERAPEUTIC TOUCH

Therapeutic touch is an ancient healing art which has recently been rediscovered. Many professionals including nurses are now incorporating it into their practice. The practitioner uses the energy field surrounding you to effect bodily changes. Practitioners teach techniques to relieve stress and pain and increase energy. One way to think of it is as a form of spiritual healing without any religious aspect.

SEX

Leaving the best to last, it has been suggested that regular sex can help reduce PMS symptoms. American reproductive biologist Winifred Cutler[6] believes that for straight women this is due to the effect of smelling a man's pheromones. Women in her trials reported that after three months of smelling their partner's armpits, periods were more regular and PMS reduced. Do bear in mind, though, that it has to be the same armpits that you are sniffing nightly – apparently, different pheromones don't have the same normalizing effect on your hormones!

Orgasms are well known for helping to relieve period pain and cramps, and for relieving stress, anxiety and low moods – perhaps a more pleasant way to use sex as a healing experience!

(For more information about alternative therapies and where you can find out about practitioners near you, see our Resources chapter.)

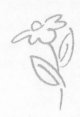

Week 11: When Temptation Strikes

Day 1

NUTRITION

Beat Your Cravings
What if you haven't stuck to the healthy eating guidelines 100 per cent?

As long as you have been doing your best and eating healthily most of the time, the occasional indulgence or setback really isn't a problem. But what if there is a time of day or an event that always ruins your healthy eating plans? For example, a leisurely dinner with friends, feeling ravenous after a workout or an attack of mid-afternoon fatigue?

Take some time today to re-read our advice on beating food cravings back on page 57. Remind yourself that if you are deficient in certain nutrients you are more likely to have cravings, so instead of reaching for junk food, reach for food that is high in magnesium (nuts, soya, green leafy veg), chromium (egg yolk, molasses, beef, hard cheese, black pepper) and B vitamins (nuts, fortified cereals, chicken, muesli, eggs).

Ward off mid-morning cravings by eating a slow-releasing energy breakfast. Start your day with wholemeal toast and Marmite, a bowl of cereal topped with chopped fruit, porridge with added sultanas or a smoothie made with yogurt, juice and fruit.

Keep healthy snacks on hand, like low-fat wholegrain crackers and hummus, vegetable juice, low-fat popcorn, fruit and a handful of nuts and seeds, hard-boiled egg, yogurt and pumpkin and sunflower seeds, or rice cakes with a thin spread of peanut butter.

EXERCISE

Quick-fix Workouts

What about those days when you just don't have 30 minutes for exercise? Here are some exercises you can do that work your entire body in only a few minutes. All you need is a little floor space.

JUMPING JACKS

Start from a standing position with your knees slightly bent. In one motion, spread your legs shoulder-width apart while swinging your arms sideways and up. Touch your hands above your head with your arms straight. Bring your feet back together and your hands to your sides. That's one. Try to do them for 2 minutes. To keep it interesting, do 10 jacks facing one direction, 10 facing another, then come back to where you started.

SKIPPING

Skipping with a rope is great fun and a good aerobic workout. Keep your shoulders relaxed and your elbows close to your body. Bend your knees slightly. Turn the rope from the wrist and try to keep a smooth arc as it passes overhead. Keep your back straight and your head up. Jump low to keep the impact on your knees and ankles to a minimum, and grip the handles lightly. Jump for 5

> minutes, and if you want, put on some upbeat music to get you in
> the mood.

Day 2

NUTRITION

Don't Let a Hangover Stop You!
You overdid it last night and your good intentions have flown out of the
window. Don't make it worse by reaching for greasy, sweet comfort foods.
Munch on some papaya and banana instead.

Papaya is a great hangover cure and will give you a lasting energy boost. A
single papaya contains all the daily recommend vitamin C. It is also rich
in natural enzymes papain and amylase, which can help settle your
stomach. Papayas also have pain-relieving properties to help ease that
thumping headache.

Banana is rich in potassium – a nutrient destroyed by alcohol. Whiz one
up into a smoothie and have a delicious drink.

EXERCISE

Quick Boosters
Some more quick-fix workouts for those days when you simply haven't
got the time for your usual 30- to 40-minute workout.

SQUAT THRUSTS

From a standing position, face a wall and place your hands on it with your feet shoulder-width apart and a few feet back from the wall. Lift one knee up towards your chest and put it down again. Then lift the other knee, and continue alternating knees for a few minutes. At first start slowly and put your feet all the way down on the floor, but then get faster, touching down only briefly on your toes.

Advanced version: Start by standing with your feet together. Then drop your knees down in front of your feet, put your weight on your hands and quickly thrust your legs straight out behind you so that you are in the plank position – like the start of a push-up. Your arms and legs are straight and your body is in one line; your weight is on your hands and feet. Then in one quick movement bring both feet back up behind your hands and return to standing. You should do the move in a rapid four counts:

1   Drop down on your hands and feet.
2   Thrust your feet out behind you.
3   Bring your feet back in.
4   Stand up and repeat.

THE WINDMILL

This exercise works your body and gives you a good stretch at the same time.

Stand up straight with your feet straight ahead, shoulder-width apart. Put your arms out to the sides with your palms down. Then bend forward at the waist and bend your knees slightly. Touch your right hand to your left toe while lifting the other arm up and over your back. Pull your left arm back to maintain a straight line with your right arm. Return to standing and repeat, but this time touch your left arm to your right toe. Think about rotating your arms like a windmill.

Day 3

NUTRITION

Car Journey Sabotage!
Another common setback to healthy eating is driving for long periods of
time. Instead of packing in junk food at a motorway service station, pack
healthy foods ahead of time. Take fruit, chopped up to make it easy to eat,
a nutritious pasta salad for an energy boost, and yogurt for slow-release
energy. Take a large bottle of water, too. Prepare a flask full of warming
herbal tea to save you from coffee made with long-life milk. And keep a
small snack, such as dried fruits or a fruit bar, in the glove compartment
of your car.

EXERCISE

Fit for Travel
If you have to travel a lot it can be tempting to let your fitness routine
slide. Don't. There are plenty of ways to stay fit when you are on the
move:

- Call the place you'll be staying and find out what facilities they have.
  Wouldn't you hate it if they had a gym and you forgot your gear?
- Bring your running shoes. One of the best ways to get to know a new
  area is on foot.
- In your hotel room you can do your toning and your stretching and the
  quick-fix workouts mentioned earlier this week.
- When flying, drink a lot of water, avoid alcohol and get out of your seat
  and walk around whenever you can, stretching your arms out in front
  of you, bending and arching your back, rolling your head and shoulders
  and rotating your ankles. You could also do your yoga breathing
  exercises.

Day 4

NUTRITION

Healthy Carry-outs
Do you often feel really ravenous after your workout? Take a post-workout snack with you to the gym. Ideally a wholemeal tuna or chicken sandwich (use a meat-substitute if you are a veggie), plus water and a sports drink if you work out for longer than two hours. Meat contains the essential acid leucine. According to US research reported in *The Journal of Nutrition*, eating leucine immediately after a workout (found in meat and dairy as well as in protein bars and some sports drinks) leads to swifter recovery.

You should also eat a small carbohydrate snack, such as a banana or a few rice cakes in the hour before you exercise to stave off hunger and fuel your workout.

EXERCISE

Boost Your Body, Unwind your Mind
Even if you hate gyms, exercise classes can be a great way to get in shape. Many classes these days encourage the mind-body-spirit connection. Eastern disciplines such as yoga and tai chi and martial arts like karate, tae kwon do, kung fu and qigong are increasingly popular. Kick-boxing aerobics is very popular these days, especially among women. It is a workout that incorporates physical elements of martial arts in a fitness class that anyone can enjoy – without having to battle an opponent.

Day 5

NUTRITION

Working Lunches
Don't skip lunch! If you really don't have time for lunch, then eat some dried fruits, nuts or a fruit-and-nut bar to stave off hunger pangs until you

can eat properly. Eating nothing will send your blood sugar plummeting and reduce your performance later in the day. Make sure you do everything you can to take a lunch break and eat a proper meal, however busy you are.

EXERCISE

Get in Balance

Practising your balance is important because it encourages you to use muscles that stabilize your body, especially those in your core. Focusing on your strong core muscles – the deepest muscle layer – as well as the superficial muscles that move your arms and legs can improve all-round strength and improve your balance and power. Spinning and step class are a good way to train your core muscles and practise your balancing skills. Dance and yoga classes are another good way to train your balancing skills.

Day 6 and 7

NUTRITION

Avoid Weekend Temptation

The weekend offers lots of temptations that can scupper your healthy diet. Here are three strategies that can help.

1 Before you go out, eat a bowl of soup to take the edge off your appetite and minimize indulging in greasy appetizers like crisps and dips. During the meal, eat slowly, aim to be one of the last people to finish your meal and take small portions. Avoid drinking wine while you are eating. Alcohol has been shown to stimulate the appetite, so wait until you have finished dinner before you have your drink.

2 Have a carbohydrate-rich comfort snack in your bag ready to eat for a night out on the town. Try a low-fat sultana muffin, a banana and a small bar of plain chocolate, peanut butter, wholemeal sandwiches or a mix of nuts, seeds and dried fruit.

3   Research shows that you are more likely to eat more if you snack or eat a meal in front of your TV. If you have a real chocolate craving, switch off the TV and indulge in a tiny portion of your desired food while completely concentrating on the taste, smell and texture. Just a mouthful eaten in this way will fulfil a craving better than bars of chocolate scarfed without thinking.

EXERCISE

Trust Yourself – Not New Trends
The search for new and exciting ways to get fit never ceases. There is disco yoga, circuit-training, basketball aerobics and trampolining, to mention but a few.

The important thing is that you find the fitness routine that suits you. Just because your friend is touting the glories of step or yoga doesn't mean you have to do it. Find something that you enjoy and benefit from. Keep looking for new ways to exercise but listen to your body, have fun and stay committed to fitness at the same time.

EMOTIONAL WELL-BEING

Discover the Positives in PMS
They do exist!

> There is a lot I hate about PMS – the mood swings, the sore breasts, the insomnia and the bloating – but there is one thing I like. For some crazy reason, a week or so before I'm due I feel really alive. I'm full of ideas, full of purpose and I want to make a difference. Somehow when my period comes I haven't got the same intensity and focus. But when I'm premenstrual I'm not content with second best – I want to be a winner.
> Lucy, 38

A 1989 study at the Canadian Well Woman Clinic revealed that seven out of ten women did have at least one positive symptom in their premenstrual phase. The study showed that women are very sensitive during this time to light, sound and smell, and women who were creative – artists, actresses, musicians – reported that they felt more creative and inspired.

This week, as the plan draws to a close and you are well on the way to seeing an improvement in your symptoms, think about anything positive that you can harness in your premenstrual phase. Here are some things you might consider:

- 31 per cent of the women in the Canadian study reported an increased enjoyment of sex.
- If problems niggling away at the back of your mind come to the fore, capitalize on your feelings of urgency and get things done. Let PMS remind you of the importance of spring-cleaning in our lives, sorting out problems and moving on.
- If you dream more in your premenstrual phase, you might want to record your dreams in your diary to increase your understanding of your character, release tension and boost your self-esteem. For example, dreaming about situations that scare you can be a good way to confront your fears. Seeing yourself cope well in a dream situation is a sign that you do have the ability to cope, for example.
- Appreciate the depth and variety of your personality. If you do feel low when PMS strikes, remind yourself that you also have a bright side to your personality. Those low moments are also part of the exciting, complex person that you are.

VITALITY BOOSTER

Take Your Mind Off PMS

My PMS is always at its worse when I'm not involved in something creative. I'm a freelance artist and most of the time I'm painting, but it's during those times when I haven't really got something to lose myself in that the tiredness really hits me and symptoms seem to bite harder.
Lori, 36

This week think of ways to nurture your creativity. Find a quiet spot sometime this week and consider these possibilities.

- Are you an artist of life – an inspired cook, a master of diplomacy, a stylish dresser? Write down all the ways you can bring beauty, harmony and flair to your surroundings.
- What would you try if you didn't care about results or your performance? Think back to your childhood: Did you enjoy banging on a drum or ballet class? How can you reconnect with that sense of fun?
- Creative people are problem-solvers. If you could clear up any issue in the world, what would it be? How would you go about it?
- Is your talent appreciating other people's creative effort? Would you enjoy it more if you had a go yourself?
- Envy can be a message from your creative core. Whose talent would you like to have? How could you develop your creativity in that area?

Week 12: Pat Yourself on the Back!

Creating Your Own Plan

Keep taking positive steps this week towards a healthy lifestyle. Enjoy
planning, shopping for and cooking your healthy menus, and don't forget
that multivitamin and -mineral and your additional calcium and
magnesium supplement every day. Make time for regular exercise and
keep thinking of ways to add spice and variety to your routine. Finally, and
perhaps most important of all, be kind to yourself: do things which make
you feel good, challenge negative thinking and get a good night's sleep.

Taking Stock

Acknowledge to yourself how you have changed and progressed since
Week 1. Notice how you are helping yourself, see how much stronger you
are, how much more self-respect, self-trust, self-love and patience with
yourself you have. Give yourself a pat on the back. Reward yourself with
something really special on the last few days of the plan. You have come a
long way in the last 12 weeks and you deserve a treat. Perhaps a holiday, a
day off, a new outfit, a celebratory meal with your friends, a gadget you
have always wanted, a party?

What if your condition still hasn't improved much, even though you have carefully followed the advice in the 12-week plan? PMS symptoms can be signs of other health conditions. Make an appointment today to see your doctor. Appendix 1 lists a number of possibilities that you may need to rule out. If anything sounds familiar, ask your doctor for advice and treatment options. You may also find the advice in the A –Z of Symptoms section helpful if certain PMS symptoms continue to bother you or pop up now and again.

In the past 12 weeks you have slowly but surely put yourself in your own good hands. Trust them, along with your body and your mind, to guide you towards improved health and well-being.

Well done!

Congratulations for having the courage, commitment, discipline and creativity to stick with the plan over the last three months. We hope that from now on you'll find health and happiness every day of every month.

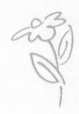

Maintenance

People ask me how I manage to be so religious about my diet and exercise. All I can say is that if a doctor gave you a prescription and told you it would save you from going mad, you would take it, wouldn't you? For me, sticking to my new routine is crucial because it has turned my life around. **Hope, 35**

The change in my diet and lifestyle has been my lifesaver. It is almost four months now and I feel so much better. My life has been transformed. My partner has come back. I am much calmer with people and don't go crazy if things go wrong. I really don't feel hopeless anymore. The real me is back and I'm going to make sure she stays. **Tamzin, 37**

Within a few months of eating healthily and exercising I was back to normal. It's amazing. My cravings disappeared and I've lost weight, too. It is five years now and I still eat as healthily as I can and make sure I exercise. I've never looked back. I'm really happy now with my life. **Lisa, 40**

Once you have completed the 12-week plan and you have noticed substantial improvements, you can then start to relax a bit. As long as you follow the 10 basic rules below, the occasional indulgence shouldn't hurt. Make sure it is only occasional to begin with – and preferably not in the run-up to your period. As a general rule, any supplements you are taking apart from your daily multivitamin and -mineral should not be necessary in the long term. They should be taken until you feel that your symptoms are well under control. This may be as little as three months or as long as nine months to a year.

You may find that weeks or months or years after the 12-week plan, PMS symptoms start to reoccur. Times of great stress or illness may place extra demands on your body and mind, and this can trigger symptoms. Should this happen, take action quickly. You can either repeat the plan to get back on track or you can identify your symptoms and take appropriate action. Again, as symptoms reduce return to the maintenance recommendations below and reduce your supplements gradually.

THE 10 BASICS

The 10 basic PMS-prevention rules below will help you keep feeling great all month long, every month:

1) EAT PLENTY OF FRUITS AND VEGETABLES
Fruit and vegetables contain a range of PMS-beating nutrients, including vitamins, mineral, antioxidants and fibre. Fresh fruits and vegetables – organic if possible – are your best option, but otherwise frozen is better than tinned if you can't get fresh.

2) EAT COMPLEX CARBS AND AVOID SIMPLE ONES
Complex carbohydrates such as brown rice, oats and wholemeal bread can stop you feeling tired, balance your blood sugar to minimize food cravings and help balance your hormones. They are also a good source of fibre, which plays an important role in balancing your hormones. With the exception of fruit (which you should always eat with some protein to slow down the effect on your blood sugar), simple carbohydrates are all refined foods from which all the nutritional goodness has been stripped away.

3) EAT LITTLE AND OFTEN

To help maintain a steady blood sugar level, aim to eat complex carbohydrates as part of your main meals and to make sure that you eat little and often during the day.

4) EAT PHYTOESTROGENS AND OILY FISH, NUTS, SEEDS AND OILS, AND MINIMIZE SATURATED FATS

Phytoestrogens have a controlling effect on your hormone levels and can be found in most vegetables and fruits. They are most beneficial in the form of legumes such as soya, lentils, chickpeas, etc. Saturated fats – found in meat and dairy products – can upset hormone balance. Eat essential fats: Omega-6 oils – found in nuts and seeds, evening primrose, starflower and borage oil – and Omega-3 – found in oily fish (tuna, mackeral, sardines, herring and salmon) and linseed oil and also in walnuts, pumpkin seed and green leafy vegetables.

5) DRINK ENOUGH WATER

Your body is around 70 per cent water, so aim to drink around six glasses of water a day to stay hydrated.

6) REDUCE YOUR INTAKE OF CASSAP

CASSAP stands for Caffeine, Alcohol, Salt, Sugar, Additives and Preservatives.

Caffeine has a diuretic effect on your body, depleting valuable stores of nutrients.

Alcohol also depletes nutrients and can upset your blood sugar balance. It also can interfere with the liver's ability to detoxify your system.

Sugar is just empty calories and is a major cause of blood sugar imbalance.

Salt can contribute to bloating, weight gain, breast tenderness and high blood pressure.

Additives, preservatives and chemicals can all contribute to hormonal imbalance. Always try to eat food in its most natural state (preferably organic) and without added chemicals in the form of preservatives, sweeteners and additives.

7) DAILY MULTIVITAMIN AND –MINERAL, CALCIUM AND MAGNESIUM EVERY DAY

Remember nutritional deficiencies, especially in the B vitamins, the antioxidant vitamins C and E, and the minerals magnesium and calcium, may either cause PMS or make it worse. Take a supplement or bone formula of a balance of calcium plus magnesium in addition to your multi.

8) EXERCISE

Try to exercise for at least 30 minutes a day five or six times a week, and make your lifestyle as active as you can. If possible try to exercise at least once or twice a week outside in the fresh air, to enjoy regular exposure to daylight.

9) REDUCE STRESS

Let go of unnecessary stress. One of the best all-round tension-relievers is exercise, but deep breathing, meditation, yoga, tai chi and prayer are also excellent ways to calm your body and mind. A good laugh, a warm bath, a massage, a walk in the countryside and anything else that helps you slow down and escape from the pressures of modern life are also highly recommended.

10) THINK POSITIVE

Every day, focus on the good things in your life. Appreciate and be grateful for all that surrounds you – your family and friends, your garden or a nearby park. Create uplifting images in your mind – walking along a sunlight sandy beach, watching a waterfall or taking a walk in a pine-scented forest.

See the recipe section (p. 309) for more ideas on healthy eating.

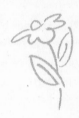

Food Sources of Essential Nutrients

Vitamin A
Vitamin A helps to fight PMS acne

Food Sources
Egg yolk, butter, milk and oily fish. Foods rich in betacarotene – the precurser of vitamin A – include red, orange and green vegetables, e.g. carrots.

Recommended Dosage for PMS
15,000 IU daily

Vitamin B Complex
Vitamin B complex is essential for stabilizing blood sugar, easing mood swings, decreasing sugar cravings, improving sleep, and fighting fatigue and headaches.

Food Sources
Whole grains, legumes and brewer's yeast, dairy produce, eggs, vegetables, fish, nuts, watermelon, avocado, seaweed

Recommended Dosage for PMS
50 to 100 mg daily

Vitamin B6
This is important for regulation of mood, memory, water balance and sleep. Several studies[1] show that B6 can reduce the discomfort associated with PMS, and that there is a link between B6 deficiency and PMS. It can ease irritability, depression, mood swings, breast tenderness, fatigue, sugar cravings, acne and water-retention.

Recommended Dosage for PMS
50-220 mg daily

Vitamin C
Vitamin C helps to fight fatigue, aches and pains, and sugar cravings. It also lessens water-retention, eases breast-swelling and boosts the immune system.

Food Sources
All fruits and vegetables, especially brussels sprouts, red peppers, citrus fruits and dark green and yellow leafy vegetables.

Recommended Dosage for PMS
500 to 1,000 mg a day

Vitamin D
This is important for energy.

Food Sources
Vitamin D-fortified margarine, eggs and oily fish are good sources. Can also be produced in the skin if it is exposed to light. Vitamin D should not be taken in large doses.

Recommended Dosage for PMS
100 IU

Vitamin E
This antioxidant is of great help easing breast tenderness. It may also relieve depression, insomnia and fatigue.[2]

Food Sources
Plant oils including sunflower and corn, and unrefined wholegrain cereals. It can also be found in sweet potatoes, asparagus, broccoli, green leafy vegetables, green beans, nuts and seeds.

Recommended Dosage for PMS
300 IU a day

Boron
Boron is essential for the efficient functioning of calcium and magnesium (two minerals important for controlling PMS). It can help ease mood swings, water-retention and sugar cravings.

Food Sources
Fruits and vegetables, especially apples, peaches, pears, grapes, legumes and peanuts

Recommended Dosage for PMS
3-9 mg daily

Calcium
Essential for growth and maintenance of healthy bones and teeth. It can also ease water-retention, mood swings, headaches and pain.

Food Sources
Dairy products, calcium-fortified soymilk, sardines, spinach, almonds and wholegrain cereals and bread

Recommended Dosage for PMS
700 mg daily

Chromium
Can help with sugar cravings and irritability, fatigue.

Food Sources
Liver, brewer's yeast, nuts and whole grains

Recommended Dosage for PMS
200-400 mg Chromium nicotinic acid complex

Iodine
Lack of iodine can result in menstrual problems and PMS fatigue.

Food Sources
Seafood, kelp, saltwater fish, seaweed, sesame seeds, soybeans and garlic

Recommended Dosage for PMS
150 mg a day

Iron
Iron is important for energy-production. One of the most common causes of fatigue is iron levels falling too low, leading to anaemia.

Food Sources
Red meat, liver, eggs, spinach and pulses

Recommended Dosage for PMS
15 mg daily

Magnesium
Magnesium deficiency has been associated with PMS. One study of magnesium levels and PMS showed a reduction in breast tenderness and bloating in 95 per cent of subjects.[3] Magnesium can help reduce water-retention and ease headaches, mood swings, sugar cravings, fatigue and low energy.

Food Sources
Wheat bran, wheatgerm, nuts, flour, dark green leafy vegetables, dried apricots, fish and tofu

Recommended Dosage for PMS
200-600 mg daily

Selenium
Lack of selenium has been linked to period problems and infertility in women.

Food Sources
Meat, fish (especially mackerel, herring and kippers) and wholemeal flour

Recommended Dosage for PMS
60-75 mcg a day

Zinc
Zinc helps to stimulate the immune system and control acne.

Food Sources
Seafood, liver, eggs, whole grains, dried beans and peas

Recommended Dosage for PMS
25-50 mg daily

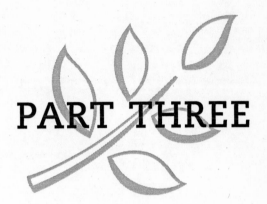

PART THREE

Fine-tuning Your Plan

What Your Doctor Can Offer You

Your doctor can offer certain prescriptions that may alleviate PMS symptoms, and we list the most common drugs below. Bear in mind that many of these drugs will concentrate on specific symptoms, such as breast tenderness or water-retention, or on manipulating your hormones to see if there is any improvement, without doing anything to address the fundamental cause of your PMS. The chances are when you stop taking the medication, symptoms will return.

One of the most interesting aspects of treating PMS with drugs is that there is a very high placebo effect. What this means is that women taking Pills which have no drugs in them (although they don't know that when they are taking them) often feel better. In every drug study there are always people who respond well to placebo, but in women with PMS over 90 per cent do. Perhaps this is because when women are given an opportunity to talk about their symptoms, have their symptoms taken seriously and take steps to improve the situation, their symptoms will improve whether they take drugs or not.

Hormonal Drugs

DANAZOL
Danazol is a synthetic hormone that suppresses ovulation, which in turn stops your periods. The theory is simple – if you are not having periods, you don't get PMS. Side-effects linked to Danazol include mood swings, nausea, dizziness and headaches, and because Danazol is a weak male hormone you may also get facial hair, acne, loss of libido, weight-gain and a deeper voice. It's up to you to decide which symptoms are worse – those of PMS or the side-effects of Danazol.

GnRH ANALOGUES
Like Danazol, GnRH stops menstruation, but it also plunges you into a temporary menopause with hot flushes, fatigue, weight-gain and night sweats.

BROMOCRIPTINE
This drug reduces high levels of prolactin in your body. Prolactin is the hormone you produce when you are breastfeeding, and bromocriptine is often prescribed for women with PMS breast pain. It won't really help any other PMS symptoms and has some unpleasant side-effects that include headaches, dizziness and vomiting.

OESTROGEN
Oestrogen patches have been shown to help women with PMS. This is basically using hormone replacement therapy (HRT) to treat PMS. If you do decide to go for this you should be aware of the risk of breast cancer associated with HRT.

PROGESTERONE
Many of the symptoms associated with PMS are thought to be linked to low progesterone levels. Dr Katharina Dalton was a pioneer in the use of progesterone therapy for women with PMS. Progesterone is normally given in the form of vaginal pessaries or skin cream. Although in this form treatment is often described as natural, the word 'natural' is

misleading as the progesterone is not the same as that produced by your ovaries. Even though some progesterone creams are synthesized from wild yam, so-called natural progesterones are drugs, not natural or herbal products.

MEFENAMIC ACID

This is a drug used to treat PMS symptoms such as headaches, mood swings and breast pain. There are uncomfortable side-effects such as indigestion, nausea, bloating, constipation and cramping.

Diuretics

Diuretics are used to help with water-retention, but they also flush out important PMS-beating nutrients such as potassium.

The Pill

We've saved the Pill to last because it is the most commonly prescribed treatment for PMS, and for some women it works. On balance, however, research[1] shows that the Pill is not an effective treatment for PMS, for the reasons outlined below.

RISKS ASSOCIATED WITH THE PILL

The Pill is an effective form of contraception, but it can also create problems such as depletion of nutrients, difficulty for some women in re-establishing a menstrual cycle or conceiving after stopping, raised blood pressure, risk of blood-clotting and a higher risk of some types of cancer.

The risks are similar for both the combined Pill (a combination of synthetic oestrogen and progesterone) and the mini-Pill (progesterone only), although the combined Pill is often thought to be more potent. Taking the combined Pill increases the risk of heart disease, particularly in women who smoke. Studies[2] in Britain reveal that a woman who is on the Pill is twice as likely to experience a fatal blood-clot as a non-Pill user. The problem is so worrying that the Family Planning Association recently launched a public education campaign to target Pill-users.

But it's the lesser-known risks of the Pill, namely blood sugar imbalance and nutritional deficiencies and how they are particularly important for women with PMS, which we'd like to draw your attention to.

The British Medical Association (BMA) lists blood sugar problems and insulin resistance as a possible side effect. 'Oestrogens may also trigger the onset of diabetes mellitus in susceptible people, or aggravate blood sugar control in diabetic women.'[3]

According to various studies,[4] the Pill can leach valuable supplements and nutrients as well as alter your vitamin and mineral levels. The studies suggest that the Pill lowers levels of:

- vitamins B1, B2 and B6 in the blood, causing hair loss, thinning hair and a decrease in progesterone
- B12, resulting in anaemia, hair loss, dry hair, brittle nails and fatigue
- Folic acid, resulting in skin discoloration,
- The antioxidants vitamins C and E, which can cause fluctuating oestrogen levels
- Zinc, which can result in acne and a decrease in oestrogen -balancing progesterone. You need sufficient levels of zinc to maintain a healthy reproductive system and hormonal balance.
- Levels of vitamin A and iron increase slightly, as do levels of copper – which isn't necessarily a good thing as high copper levels can increase the risk of high blood pressure.

The Pill can also kill friendly bacteria in your gut, which can cause digestive problems. If you are taking the Pill, live yogurt, which contains natural probiotics, should be on your daily menu to restore the bacterial balance. If you are dairy intolerant you can buy fruit-based drinks with live bacterial cultures from healthfood shops. The Pill can also lower levels of good cholesterol, and increases levels of bad cholesterol, so you need to ensure that you eat to prevent heart disease.

THE PILL AND DIETARY SUPPLEMENTS

Vitamin A
High levels of vitamin A have been found in women who take the Pill, so if you are on the Pill it isn't a good idea to supplement with vitamin A.

Vitamin C
Concern that vitamin C increases the effectiveness of oestrogen – and as oestrogen has been linked with PMS symptoms, and an excess relative to progesterone can trigger dizziness and forgetfulness, and has also been linked, in the form of HRT, with increased risk of breast cancer – has led one group of experts to caution women Pill-users against taking vitamin C supplements. An investigation,[5] however, showed that taking 1g of vitamin C a day does not raise oestrogen levels in women on the Pill.

B Vitamins
If you are on the Pill you are likely to be deficient in B vitamins, which help your liver break down hormones, so it is wise to supplement with extra B vitamins.

Vitamin K
When on the Pill supplementing with K vitamins should be avoided, since vitamin K is involved with the risk of blood-clotting, and the risk of blood clots is increased by synthetic hormones already. Dietary intake of vitamin K – found in green vegetables and cauliflower – need not be restricted.

Copper and Zinc
Higher levels of copper are associated with Pill use. Copper competes with zinc, which is essential for women with PMS. So it is best to avoid any supplements containing copper.

The health risks associated with being on the Pill increase dramatically if you are overweight or if you smoke. The better and more permanent solution is to make healthy diet and lifestyle changes, with or without medication.

FINDING THE RIGHT PILL

If you are aware of the risks and still want to stay on the Pill for the time being, you need to find the Pill that best suits your individual needs.

Oral contraceptives come in two basic types – oestrogen containing combined and phased oral contraceptives, and progesterone-only contraceptives. The combined oral contraceptive Pill is the most widely prescribed because it is the most reliable.

Progesterone-only Pills are slightly less reliable and must be taken at exactly the same time each day to have an effect. Some women also find that progesterone-only Pills, or Pills with low doses of oestrogen, seem to make their PMS symptoms worse.

- You are less likely to experience breast tenderness with Marvelon, Minulet, Femodene, Microgynon or Ovranette.
- Headaches can be made worse with water-retention, common with more oestrogenic Pills. You are less likely to experience headaches and migraines with Microgynon and Ovranette.
- You are less likely to experience water-retention and weight-gain with Pills containing the modern progesterones, such as Femodene.
- You are less likely to experience excess hair with Dianette or Cilest.
- If taking the Pill seems to affect your libido, try Ovysmen, Brevinor, Femodene, Minulet or Mercillon
- If you are prone to acne, the progesterone in the Pill may make it worse. Try Minulet, Femodene, Ovysmen or Brevinor, which are less likely to cause acne. Dianette is actually licensed as a treatment for acne.

The best advice is to proceed with caution if you are taking oral contraceptives, and to monitor things carefully. If you think the Pill is making you feel worse, tell your doctor straight away. You may also find that after taking a brand of Pill for several months or even years you start getting symptoms of PMS. This could be a result of blood sugar imbalance.

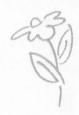

A-Z of PMS Symptoms and
How to Beat Them

You may find that while your body becomes healthier and more balanced when you are on the plan, or immediately after finishing it, certain symptoms still surface from time to time. If this is the case, this A to Z of the most common PMS symptoms can help. Pick and choose the remedies that cater to your particular PMS symptoms, and fine-tune the 12-week plan to suit your needs.

Acne/ Spots

According to Anthony Chu, Senior Dermatologist at the Imperial College of Science, Technology and Medicine, Hammersmith Hospital in London, the cause of spots isn't chocolate, fatty food, cakes, sweets or poor hygiene, although these won't help the condition. It's an increase in the skin's production of oil, called sebum.

Oestrogen helps to regulate sebum, but in the run-up to your period oestrogen levels fall and more sebum is produced. Androgen hormones – of which testosterone is the most well known – increase the production of sebum. In women who get spots only in the run-up to a period, it is thought that for some reason the adrenal glands may be producing too much androgen hormone.

The typical treatment offered for spots is antibiotics, but this isn't a good idea if you have PMS. They won't help address the real cause of the problem and are likely to increase the risk of Candida. If you do suffer from bouts of premenstrual spots, keep your blood sugar levels in balance and control stress so that your adrenal glands can function normally.

DIET

It is especially important that you include plenty of phytoestrogens in your diet (see page 22). Phytoestrogens can help your body control the amount of testosterone circulating in your blood.

Vitamin B6[1] has been shown to be beneficial for PMS spots. Foods rich in B6 include bananas, fish, lean meat, nuts, seeds and wholegrains.

Make sure you get your essential fatty acids. Flaxseed oil and primrose oil are good sources of the essential fatty acids needed to keep skin smooth and clear.

Limit your intake of alcohol, sugar, processed food, salt, butter, caffeine, chocolate, eggs, fried foods, meat, margarine, wheat, soft drinks and food containing hydrogenated vegetable oils.

To ease inflammation or prevent infection, eat lots of garlic. Garlic is a powerful antibiotic. Grate it on your food or take it as a supplement every day. This will also help protect your heart.

Women with PMS can be deficient in zinc, and zinc is important for hormonal balance. It is also helpful for keeping testosterone and acne flare-ups in check. Make sure you are getting enough zinc in your diet, found in foods such as shellfish, soybeans and sunflower seeds, or take 30 mg a day of zinc supplement for two to three months.

Eating sulphur-rich foods such as eggs and onions can also help, and live yogurt with bifidus and acidophilus bacteria rebalance the bacteria in your gut and protect against inflammation.

HELPING YOURSELF
Regular exercise is helpful because it encourages hormonal balance and healthy blood flow to your face to help flush out toxins.

Keep make-up to a minimum and cleanse thoroughly with a mild – but not astringent – skincare product. Never leave make-up on at night, and choose oil-free moisturizers and make-up. Opt for loose rather than pressed powders, and powder blushes instead of creams. Look for the word 'non-comedogenic' on labels.

Always try to cleanse your skin twice a day, but don't use harsh cleansers or toners with alcohol – these strip the skin of natural oils, encouraging it to produce more in response, and increase the chance of spots.
Avoid abrasive scrubs. They can cause infection and make acne worse. Use one specifically recommended by a dermatologist if you use one at all. Never pick or squeeze spots – this can cause scarring.

Dabbing vitamin E oil on acne scars can help them to heal. Pierce a capsule of vitamin E with a pin and squeeze the oil out to apply it. If you suffer primarily from blackheads, Retinol, a vitamin A derivative, softens and expels them and can help to prevent inflammation.

NATURAL TREATMENTS
Tea-tree oil has good antiseptic, anti-bacterial and anti-fungal properties. Dab it onto your spots. A study conducted by the Department of Dermatology of the Royal Prince Alfred Hospital in New South Wales, Australia, found a 5 per cent solution of tea tree oil was as effective as a 5 per cent solution of benzoyl peroxide for most cases of acne, and had no side-effects. Use a tea tree moisturizer.

There are a number of homeopathic remedies for acne – Nux Vomica, Pulsatilla and Hepar Sulph, for example. If you aren't sure about a homeopathic remedy straight from the shelf, consult a qualified practitioner.

Ketsugo is made from isolutrol, a substance originally derived from shark's bile but now synthesized. It's rich in antioxidants and, according to Dr David Fenton from St John's Department of Dermatology at St Thomas's Hospital in London, it appears to be able to regulate the production of sebum and soften the skin.

Pure aloe vera gel is antibacterial and soothing. Some women find that dabbing it on their acne every day really helps.

For angry, inflamed spots or acne, witch hazel is cooling and soothing. Dab directly on the acne.

Echinacea is one of nature's most powerful antibiotics. Dab a tincture or cream on the affected skin daily.

If your doctor tells you that you have higher-than-normal androgen levels, the herb saw palmetto can work as an anti-androgen and this can be helpful for premenstrual acne. Perhaps the most helpful herb though is Agnus Castus (see page 238), which has been found to be beneficial in the treatment of PMS acne. Other beneficial herbs include burdock root, red clover and milk thistle, which are powerful blood-cleansers. All these should be prescribed by a medical herbalist.

Light therapy, which involves shining different types of light on the acne, from UV to simply coloured light, can help. Red lights have been shown to open capillaries and boost circulation, while blue light closes them. Ask a dermatologist for advice.

Bloating

Over-the-counter remedies aren't really a good idea, as they can leach valuable nutrients from your body, but if you do get fluid retention there are a number of things you can do to help yourself.

DIET

Cut down on your salt intake. Use less salt in your cooking, watch out for hidden salts in your foods, and look for other ways to enhance flavour (see pages 22–3).

Increase your fluid intake. You need to drink more, not less, to help your body dilute the salt in your tissues and allow you to excrete more salt and fluid. Aim to drink at least 2 to 3 litres of water a day.

Reduce the amount of caffeine in your diet. Caffeine is a diuretic, but it won't ease bloating because it hinders the secretion of excess salt and toxins from your body

Eat more potassium-rich foods to bring down your body's sodium level, as the two minerals balance each other out. Reach for those bananas, apricots, black beans, lentils, tomatoes, green leafy vegetables and fresh fruits.

Make sure your diet includes sufficient B vitamins, especially vitamin B6 – found in bananas, lean meat, fish, nuts, seeds and wholegrains – which is a tried-and-tested remedy for PMS water-retention.

Eat foods that naturally decrease fluid-retention, like asparagus, apple cider vinegar, alfalfa sprouts and dandelion flowers.

Keep your blood sugar levels in balance. When blood sugar levels drop adrenaline is released to move sugar quickly from your cells into your blood. When the sugar leaves the cells it is replaced by water, which contributes to that bloated feeling.

NATURAL THERAPIES

Studies at the University of Reading have shown the surprising effectiveness of Colladeen, a mix of grapeseed extract, bilberry and cranberry extract, for relief of PMS bloating.

Aromatherapy oils can be helpful with bloating. Add juniper, fennel or camomile to a warm bath and soak for 20 minutes, or use one of these as a massage oil.

Homeopathic remedies, especially Natrum Nur, can help with water-retention. Ask a medical herbalist for advice.

Dandelion and parsley are natural herbal diuretics packed with PMS-beating nutrients that allow fluid to be released without losing nutrients.

Elevate your feet if you are prone to swelling in the ankles. And wear supportive stockings to ease discomfort.

If bloating is due to constipation, see the section on Digestive Problems (page 288).

Breast Tenderness

Some women experience such breast tenderness that they can't bear to be touched or hugged, and find it hard to sleep because they can't find a comfortable position. Make sure you wear a comfortable, supportive bra – one that does not irritate the nipple area as you move. Then try the recommendations below. You might initially consider a nonprescription pain-reliever such as aspirin or ibuprofen. (Most breast pain is not linked to severe health conditions like cancer, but never ignore the pain. Any unusual changes should be reported to your doctor.)

DIET
Studies[2] have shown that women who live in Asian countries don't have the same degree of breast discomfort, and diet is the crucial factor here. The diet of most Asian women tends to rely less on processed and fatty foods. So the first step is to eat healthily according to the 12-week plan.

Make sure you get your phytoestrogens, found in foods such as soya, chickpeas and lentils. The diet of Asian women is high in phytoestrogens, which help keep hormones in balance.

Cut down on foods and drinks containing caffeine. They have been shown to increase problems with tender breasts.

Up your fibre intake. Research[3] has shown that there may be a link between constipation and a painful breast condition called fibrocystic breast disease. So make sure you drink enough water and have a good intake of fibre to ensure regularity. You may also like to sprinkle some flaxseed on your cereal in the morning. Don't, however, include bran in your diet. Bran can make things worse because it contains substances called phytates, which can interfere with the absorption of important PMS-beating nutrients, like magnesium and calcium.

Vitamin E has been shown[4] to reduce breast pain and tenderness in many studies. Eat foods rich in vitamin E such as oats, sunflower oil, whole grains, soya oil and leafy green vegetables. You may also like to take a supplement for a couple of months to give you a kick-start.

Eat some live yogurt every day. Breast tenderness may be related to an excess of oestrogen, and the beneficial bacteria in live yogurt can help to reabsorb old hormones and also to increase the efficiency of your bowel movements.

Increase your intake of Omega-3 fatty acids. Omega-3 fatty acids, found in fish oil, have been found to relieve breast tenderness and fluid-retention. Take fish oil capsules, eat more fish, or sprinkle linseeds and hemp seeds on to your salads and soups.

The B vitamins are of particular value if you suffer from breast tenderness because they help your liver break down excess oestrogen. Improve your intake of B vitamin foods (see pages 267–8), and think about taking a B complex supplement for a couple of months.

NATURAL THERAPIES

Older studies[5] showed that supplementing your diet with evening primrose oil, which contains GLA (gamma linoleic acid), could reduce breast discomfort. More recent studies do not show this correlation. The only way to find out if it can help you is trial and error. The suggested dosage is between 240 and 320 mg a day. Do bear in mind though that evening primrose oil needs to be taken for about three months to be effective, so stick with it.

A number of essential aromatherapy oils, such as lavender, fennel and juniper, can encourage lymphatic drainage and help relieve breast pain by helping to regulate hormones. Massage the oil on your breasts, putting one drop of your chosen oil in a teaspoon of carrier oil such as sweet almond or sunflower, or use a few drops in your bath.

Homeopathic remedies such as Lachesis, Pulsatilla and Natrum Nur may also prove useful. Ask a homeopath for advice.

The herb Ginkgo Biloba has proved to be effective according to a French study[6] where women with PMS breast tenderness taking Ginko Biloba reported less pain than those taking a placebo. Other helpful herbs include Agnus Castus to balance hormones and milk thistle to help your liver process oestrogen efficiently, allowing excess to be excreted. Ask a medical herbalist for advice.

Digestive Problems

Digestive problems in the run-up to a period can include diarrhoea, constipation and nausea.

DIET
Increase the amount of fibre in your diet (see pages 118–19). This will create bulk in your intestines and ensure regular bowel movements.

Make sure you drink plenty of water. Drinking hot water with lemon juice in the morning will encourage regular bowel movements.

Peppermint and fennel teas after a meal can ease bloating and reduce trapped wind.

If you have diarrhoea avoid alcohol, caffeine, milk and dairy products until the diarrhoea has subsided. Try some potassium-rich banana, applesauce, rice and dry toast until you feel better to help restore balance to your body. You can also use live yogurt to replace beneficial bacteria in your intestines. Don't take any anti-diarrhoeal medications until you have given these recommendations a chance to work.

HELPING YOURSELF
Chew your food slowly and thoroughly to encourage proper digestion. Before you begin a meal, start with a few cleansing breaths and breathe fully as you eat. Try to avoid distractions when you eat, like the TV.

If you have intestinal cramping and gas all month long in spite of these remedies, you may have irritable bowel syndrome, which is a disorder that needs medical attention.

If you get nausea along with digestive distress, try drinking camomile tea three times a day. Vitamin B6 can help quell nausea. Increase the amount in your diet or take a supplement. Ginger is also great for easing nausea. Brew a cup of ginger tea and drink daily. If stomach acid is a problem, a cup of licorice root tea has been shown to be effective.

Acupressure has been found to be effective for reducing nausea. You can purchase acupressure bands (worn around your wrists) in many chemists.

DISORIENTATION AND CLUMSINESS
Studies[7] show that in the premenstrual period the nervous system is affected, and this can cause lack of coordination, poor concentration and clumsiness. The exact cause is unknown.

Difficulty concentrating and becoming absent-minded may be related to fluid-retention, lack of sleep and stress.

DIET

Pay particular attention to eating little and often and cutting down on caffeine to ensure that your nervous system isn't being overworked by too much adrenaline.

Make sure that your diet is sufficient in B vitamins – especially vitamin B5, found in foods such as whole grains, whole rice, wholemeal bread, legumes, broccoli and tomatoes. Vitamin B5 is essential for optimum functioning of your nervous system.

If lack of co-ordination is a real problem you may want to supplement with an additional 50 mg of vitamin B5 a day on top of your multivitamin and -mineral.

Ensure that your diet is sufficient in magnesium (see pages 270–1), which can help control the stress response.

Make sure your diet is sufficient in iron (see page 270). Low iron levels can be associated with memory problems and poor coordination.

HELPING YOURSELF

Learn a relaxation technique like that on page 92, to give your nervous system a chance to repair and relax. Just a few minutes a day of relaxation is enough.

Practise yoga and meditation to help improve concentration and awareness (see pages 107–8, 172).

Research has shown that Gingko Bilboa can improve concentration, memory and reaction time. Gingko helps deliver oxygen to your nerve cells and your brain. A study in the *Lancet*[8] showed that Gingko can improve blood flow to the head. If mental and/or physical disorientation is a problem you may want to take a tincture of Gingko for a period of three to four months. Remember, herbs take a few weeks of daily use to create improvement.

Homeopathic remedies, such as Sepia, Pulsatilla, Lycopodium and Natrum Nur, may prove useful. Ask at your pharmacy for advice.

Try some essential oils to soothe your mind and body and reduce unhelpful stress. Melissa, lavender and camomile all have a calming effect which can help problems that contribute to clumsiness.

Review the information in the 12-week plan if you suspect your disorientation has anything to do with fatigue (see below – if you aren't getting quality sleep, memory will be affected), anxiety, stress and depression or feeling out of control (see pages 78–108).

Dry Skin

Dermatitis and eczema – both of which can cause itching – can occur in the run-up to a period. Itching typically occurs on the hands, face, scalp and behind the knees, and can increase with stress.

First check that you don't have any allergic reaction to the foods you are eating or the substances that come into contact with your skin, such as washing powder. Then consider these remedies to reduce your discomfort:

- Try using a cortisone cream or lotion or a calamine-type lotion.
- Cool compresses or a washcloth soaked in milk and water can help.
- Apply cooled camomile tea to the skin with a soft cloth.
- Talk yourself out of scratching, and use breathing and relaxation strategies for reducing stress (as outlined in the 12-week plan) to resist the urge.
- Keep your fingernails short, smooth and clean.

Fatigue

Fatigue is perhaps the most common symptom of PMS – you just don't feel you have your usual stamina. The Vitality Boosters in the 12-week plan and the information on beating PMS-related fatigue on pages 206–8 are all designed to help boost your energy levels. So use that information to focus in on this problem if you find you just can't shake it off.

Headaches

Headaches come in many different varieties. The most usual for women with PMS are the tension-type and sinus headaches. It is interesting that many women who get migraines stop having headaches when they fall pregnant, so the link between headaches and hormonal change is clear.

DIET

The best solution in the long term is to eat the hormone- and blood sugar-regulating diet recommended by the 12 week-plan. Missing meals can trigger a headache whether you are premenstrual or not.

See if you can find a pattern or a trigger to your headaches. When you get a headache, note what you've eaten, when you've eaten and how you felt when you ate. Perhaps you are sensitive to certain foods when you are premenstrual. Watch out especially for foods such as cheese, red wine, chocolate, citrus juice or fruit, which contain tyramine, phenylethylamine and histamine – all of which can trigger headaches.

Unfortunately, symptoms often don't hit you immediately after eating, so you may need to keep a diary for several weeks to notice a pattern.

Magnesium helps your muscles to relax, and a deficiency can trigger headaches. So make sure your diet includes foods such as leafy green vegetables, nuts and seeds, bitter chocolate, soya beans and whole grains. One study[9] showed that women who took 300 mg of magnesium twice a day reported fewer headaches than those who did not.

Make sure your diet is rich in essential fatty acids – especially Omega-3. Another study[10] showed that migraine sufferers showed a significant reduction in symptoms when they took Omega-3 fish oils every day.

HELPING YOURSELF

It's best to avoid over-the-counter painkillers, as many contain caffeine and you can also develop an intolerance to them.

Track your headaches and try to pinpoint the factors that trigger them. Typical tension headache-triggers include stress, fatigue, too much sleep, lack of exercise, and activities that require repetitive motion such as chewing gum or grinding teeth. Migraines can be triggered by certain foods and drinks, or they can be hormonally triggered by perimenopause or the use of oral contraceptives, lack of sleep, bright lights, weather changes, stress and strong smells.

Learn to relax. By reducing muscle tension you may be able to ward off a fair number of headaches. Sit or lie down in a dark, quiet room for 20 minutes. Place an ice pack on your forehead. Tension headaches sometimes respond better to the application of heat.

Regular exercise and stretching can prevent many tension headaches. Perform stretching exercises for your neck, shoulders and back a few times a day. If you also get back or joint pain, pay attention to your posture throughout the day (see pages 154–7).

Do your yoga breathing exercises to increase the flow of blood, oxygen and glucose to your brain, and to improve your circulation (see pages 157–8).

Treat yourself to a neck, shoulder and head massage. Whether it is a traditional massage or acupressure, releasing physical tension and improving circulation can promote feelings of well-being and even prevent headaches. Simply rubbing your temples can relieve pain.

Use a blend of relaxing aromatherapy oils as a massage oil, or add a few drops in your bath. Lavender, camomile and rosemary can all ease pain.

A homeopath will look at your diet and lifestyle and suggest an individual remedy according to your symptoms. Most commonly used remedies for acute headaches include Natrum Nur, Belladonna, Aconite, Hypericum, Nux Vomica, Pulsatilla, Bryonia and Lycopodium. Ask a qualified homeopath or your pharmacist for advice.

Many women find that acupuncture is a useful treatment for headaches and migraines.

A warm bath, or just putting your feet in warm water, may offer relief. If you also get pain in your joints, a hot bath for about 30 minutes will help increase blood flow to the joints. If you get premenstrual cramps, a hot bath or hot-water bottle can also help.

If you have a tension headache and can't get to a dark room to relax, put your hands around the back of your head and drop your chin on your chest. Press your chin down and hold for a minute. Then use your hands to turn your head to the right and hold for a minute. Then back to the centre and hold for a minute, then to the left and then back to centre, again for a minute each time.

One study[11] showed that 70 per cent of migraine sufferers had less frequent attacks when taking the herb feverfew. The herb milk thistle may also be beneficial, as it helps to improve liver function.

Don't ignore headaches that occur over and over again. They could be a sign of an underlying health problem. If you have tried various DIY measures or your headaches become more intense or persistent, ask your doctor for advice.

Mood Swings

DIET

Mood swings are classic signs of low blood sugar, so eat healthy and nutritious meals and snacks throughout the day. Don't go for long periods without food. And avoid caffeine and foods packed with sugar.

Consider taking a B vitamin supplement, magnesium supplement and Omega-3 fish oil supplement in addition to your multivitamin and -mineral. B vitamins can help your body produce serotonin, which is the feel-good hormone. Magnesium is well known as 'nature's tranquillizer', and essential fatty acids are important for hormonal balance.

HELPING YOURSELF

Try some Siberian Ginseng to help boost your adrenal glands and help you deal with stress.

There are lots of homeopathic remedies for mood swings:

- Pulsatilla   When you feel sad for no reason
- Lycopodium   When you feel depressed
- Causticum   When you feel irritable and sensitive
- Sepia   When you feel weepy and chilly, and crave sweet foods
- Nux vomica   When you feel irritable and constipated.

Ask your homeopathic pharmacist for advice.

Try aromatherapy oils in a massage or a bath, such as relaxing lavender, mood-enhancing camomile and rose oil, or calming sandalwood and clary sage.

Try some cognitive behavioural therapy anger-management strategies if you are prone to angry outbursts. Remind yourself that you do have some control over yourself despite the way you are feeling. Question your motives. When you feel angry, stop and ask yourself why you feel this way and if your anger is appropriate to the situation. If you can do something positive, do it. If you can't do anything then it is time to use your breathing, meditation and relaxation techniques to chill out. Find ways to release your anger by either confronting someone calmly to make your point or using a punchbag or going for a brisk walk. Write in your emotions diary and try to see patterns to your feelings and behaviour.

For more advice and helpful strategies on how to deal with anger, see pages 146–8. For depression, see page 299, and for mood swings, see pages 141–2.

Mouth Ulcers or Canker Sores

DIET

Deficiencies in iron, B12 and folic acid have been linked to painful mouth ulcers. Vitamin C and zinc are also important because they can enhance immune function and aid wound-healing. Other helpful strategies include: Good dental hygiene – yes, you do need to floss every day.

Eat plenty of salad with raw onions. Onions contain sulphur, which has healing properties.

- Avoid sugar, citrus fruits and refined, processed foods.
- Avoid chewing gum, lozenges, sharp sweets, mouthwashes, tobacco, coffee, citrus fruits and any other food which may trigger these sores.
- Consult your GP if you have a mouth sore that does not heal.
- Stress and allergies are perhaps the most common triggers for mouth sores, so pay attention to your stress levels as recommended throughout the 12-week plan.
- You can buy gel-like ointment from your chemist – like bonjela – that is applied directly to the ulcer. It sticks to the sore and provides relief.

Night Sweats

Night sweats or hot flushes may not be associated with the perimenopause but with PMS. Body temperature changes can be stimulated by the drop in ovarian hormones just before a period. Avoid alcohol, spicy foods and hot baths to minimize potential triggers. And check out the remedies for sleep problems referred to above. If the problem happens all month long or increases in intensity and frequency, consult your doctor to see if they are related to the perimenopause.

Sleep Problems

Whether you have problems falling asleep, staying asleep, waking up or sleeping too much, you can benefit from some basic sleep-hygiene routines. These include sticking to a regular sleeping and waking routine, avoiding or cutting down on food, caffeine, alcohol and exercise a few hours before bed, getting daily exercise and exposure to daylight, and making sure your bedroom is a good environment for sleep.

Sugar Cravings

Eat little and often and reduce your intake of caffeine and sugar to keep your blood sugar levels in balance. Then put yourself in a calmer frame of mind with meditation or relaxation exercises to help you control bingeing.

The most important natural therapies for sugar and food cravings are chromium and the herb Garcinia cambognia. Foods rich in chromium include liver, mushrooms, wholegrains and yeast.

If you don't suffer from diabetes, you may want to think about taking a Garcinia or chromium supplement for a few months until the cravings disappear. Garcinia contains substances which can control appetite. It also helps your body use carbohydrates for energy rather than for fat. Some health companies sell chromium and Garcinia tablets, but avoid Garcinia if you are prone to migraines and headaches.

Homeopathic remedies such as Sepia and Nux Vomica may also help control food cravings. Check with a qualified homeopath.

If these DIY techniques don't help, you may want to consider asking your doctor or a nutritionist for advice, or join a supervised dietary programme.

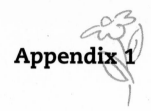

Appendix 1

Could There Be Another Cause?

Painful Periods (Dysmenorrhoea)
Unlike PMS, dysmenorrhoea occurs at the beginning of the menstrual period and during it. The most prominent symptom is severe cramping or pain in the lower abdomen or pelvic area, but it can also cause headaches, backache and nausea. If you think you have dysmenorrhoea, your first port of call should be your GP who can offer advice, information and, if needed, medication to ease the discomfort.

Endometriosis
Endometriosis occurs when pieces of the endometrium (lining of uterus) break off, escape from the uterus and become implanted on other organs, such as the ovaries, fallopian tubes and uterus. The uterine cells mimic the menstrual cycle by thickening and bleeding, but because the cells are attached to other organs, the blood has nowhere to go.

Endometriosis can cause pain before a period but, unlike PMS, the pain continues during a period. The stray cells eventually form blood blisters, scars and sometimes adhesions (abnormal scar tissue that holds the organs together). These scars and adhesions can cause problems with fertility.

There are various options for endometriosis. Talk to your GP. Information and advice about lifestyle changes and websites/support groups are listed in the Resources chapter.

Pelvic Inflammatory Disease

Pelvic inflammatory disease (PID) is a term used to describe infections of any of the reproductive organs of the pelvis. In the acute or early phase the pain of PID can be severe; in the later stages the pain may be similar to PMS with lower abdominal aches and backache. An unpleasant discharge may accompany PID along with chills, fever and urinary problems. If you are experiencing any of these symptoms, consult your doctor.

Pelvic Pain

You may experience pelvic pain about seven to ten days before your period. There may also be symptoms similar to PMS, such as insomnia or headaches, but in addition there may be pain when sitting and standing. Ask your GP for advice.

Depression

Depression is an overwhelming sad feeling that does not go away – not even when good things happen or your period starts. The following are common symptoms of depression:

- loss of interest in formerly pleasurable activities
- loss of energy
- sleep disorders
- difficulty concentrating
- feelings of despair and hopelessness
- problems with food – eating too much or too little.

If you have some of these symptoms, don't use PMS as an excuse – talk to a friend, a counsellor or a doctor straight away.

Stress

If you are under stress – for example pressure at work, arguments with the kids, financial worries – this can manifest in symptoms which resemble PMS such as headaches, fatigue and irritability. The difference is that, unless the source of your stress isn't dealt with, that stressed-out feeling doesn't go away when your period comes.

If you do feel that your life is spinning out of control, consult your GP.

Perimenopause

The perimenopause is a transition stage between fertility and the menopause when a woman's rate of ovulation gradually slows down (until it stops completely at the menopause). Many of the symptoms are the same: bloating, weight gain, food cravings, headaches, depression, irritability and lack of energy and loss of concentration. You can make a quick judgement about what may be causing your symptoms with the following rule: If your periods continue to occur regularly, it's PMS. If your periods are irregular, it's the perimenopause or some other hormonal imbalance, such as PCOS (see below).

It's important to remember that the perimenopause isn't an illness. It is a perfectly natural state for your body to be in. The 12-week plan isn't tailor-made for the perimenopause, but it can encourage the kind of positive lifestyle changes that can ease symptoms.

PCOS

PCOS, or Polycystic Ovary Syndrome, is a health condition linked with hormone imbalance and insulin resistance which can bring about a raft of symptoms, from irregular or absent periods to acne, weight gain, fatigue, depression, excess body and facial hair, diabetes and hair loss. It is thought that one in ten women has this condition even though many of them may not know it because their symptoms have been misdiagnosed as PMS or stress.

If you experience any of the following, the chances are you could have PCOS:

- Do you have irregular or absent periods?
- Do you have excess facial or body hair?
- Do you get acne?
- Do you have problems with managing your weight?
- Are there problems with fertility?

If you suspect that you have PCOS, see your doctor and read the books recommended in our Suggested Reading list, which will give you information and advice about how you can manage the condition.

Candida

Everybody's gut contains *Candida albicans*, a yeast which, along with several other thousand bacteria in the gut, produces energy and other beneficial substances. Some women suffer from an overgrowth of Candida which manifests itself as vaginal or oral thrush. It is especially common when taking antibiotics, eating a lot of dairy products and if you are generally run-down. Along with thrush, other symptoms include food cravings, fatigue, headaches, bloating and a feeling of being spaced out.

A bout of oral or vaginal thrush should always be checked out by your doctor. There are plenty of other viral or bacterial causes and thrush can be aggravated by depression, irritable bowel and anaemia. If you do have an overgrowth of Candida, you may need to use a vaginal cream prescribed by a doctor. You will also need to reduce the quantity of dairy products and yeast-containing and -producing foods in your diet, and eat some live yogurt containing beneficial bacteria (*lactobacillus*, *bifidus*) every day.

Thyroid Problems

The thyroid is situated in your neck and helps to control your metabolism and body temperature. Poor thyroid function can cause symptoms similar to those of PMS, so a thyroid diagnosis may be missed. Symptoms include weight gain, feeling cold, constipation, depression, poor concentration, dry hair, hair loss, low energy, headaches and fertility problems. It is important that your thyroid is checked, as one study[1] found that if women have both PMS and thyroid problems, treating the thyroid will alleviate the PMS.

Diabetes/Blood Sugar Problems

You know how important it is to balance your blood sugars if you have PMS. Left unchecked, blood sugar problems can lead to diabetes – and many of the symptoms of diabetes are similar to those of PMS. If you are experiencing symptoms such as frequent urination, excessive thirst or increased appetite, it is important that you see your doctor to rule out diabetes and get advice about diet and treatment options.

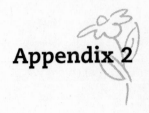

Appendix 2

Daily Records and Wall Charts

Daily Symptom Diary

Here is a week's worth of daily symptom diaries – please feel free to copy it out or photocopy it, adding your own notes, additions or artwork if you want, to make it your unique, individual record of your progress.

WEEK # ...

DAY 1

Date..........................

Medication...

Symptoms..

....

....

What did I eat today?

....

....

....

What exercise did I do?

....

....

....

Comments for today

....

....

....

Overall daily rating:

....

DAY 2

Date..........................

Medication..

Symptoms...

....

....

What did I eat today?

....

....

....

What exercise did I do?

....

....

....

Comments for today

....

....

....

Overall daily rating:

....

DAY 3

Date..........................

Medication..

Symptoms...

....

....

What did I eat today?

....

....
....

What exercise did I do?
....
....
....

Comments for today
....
....
....

Overall daily rating:
....

DAY 4
Date........................
Medication..
Symptoms..
....
....

What did I eat today?
....
....
....

What exercise did I do?
....
....
....

Comments for today
....
....
....

Overall daily rating:
....

DAY 5

Date.........................

Medication...

Symptoms...

....

....

What did I eat today?

....

....

....

What exercise did I do?

....

....

....

Comments for today

....

....

....

Overall daily rating:

....

DAY 6

Date.........................

Medication...

Symptoms...

....

....

What did I eat today?

....

....

....

What exercise did I do?

....

....

....

Comments for today

....

....

....

Overall daily rating:

....

DAY 7

Date..........................

Medication..

Symptoms..

....

....

What did I eat today?

....

....

....

What exercise did I do?

....

....

....

Comments for today

....

....

....

Overall daily rating:

....

Monthly PMS Wall Chart

You may want to make three copies of this – one to use right now, one for 'his and hers' and one if you want to repeat the plan later as a 'booster'.

Month #1	Month #2	Month #3	Month #4
1			
2			
3			
4			
5			
6			
7			
8			
9			
10			
11			
12			
13			
14			
15			
16			
17			
18			
19			
20			
21			
22			
23			
24			
25			
26			
27			
28			
29			
30			
31			

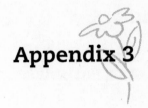

Appendix 3

PMS-busting Recipes

We do hope you enjoy experimenting with the recipes below. Many of them were submitted by women who like to cook for themselves and their families. They are quick and made with readily-available PMS-busting ingredients. You won't find any complicated recipes or ingredients here – most have fewer than 10 ingredients.

If you get into the cooking mood, you may want to invest in one or two of the many healthy-eating cookbooks available at bookshops and healthfood shops. We particularly recommend *PMS: Recipes for Health* by Jill Davies, as listed in our Suggested Reading chapter (recipes marked with an asterisk [*] have been adapted from *PMS: Recipes for Health*).

Don't forget that healthy living magazines such as *Here's Health* in the UK and *Healthy Woman* in the US often offer tips for healthy eating. Why not find or invent more healthy recipes to add to this collection here? You may even want to get a notebook or recipe file together and start your own collection.

Unless stated otherwise, all recipes serve one person.

JUICES

APPLE AND CARROT

4 carrots
1 apple

This is a basic juice that can be used as a springboard for experimentation. Once you are happy with the carrot and apple proportions (you may prefer more carrot to apple or vice versa), you can start adding other ingredients, for example, ginger, spinach or grapefruit.

APPLE, PEAR AND BERRY

2 apples
1 pear
A dozen berries

Keep a few pieces of apple to put through the juicer last. This will help flush the thicker berry juice through the machine.
Apples and pears taste sublime when juiced together. Berries are packed with nutrients, especially potassium, and any berry – strawberry, raspberry, blackberries – works well with apple and pear.

APPLE, WATERCRESS AND LEMON

2 apples
Half a lemon
As much watercress as you want to use

This is a great breakfast-time drink that really wakes your whole system up for the day.

FRUIT MEDLEY

Half a peeled apple
Half a peeled pear
1 tangerine
12 grapes
1 peach

This is a great fruit punch; the recipe can be varied and different fruits used to suit the season.

SMOOTHIES

BANANA AND PINEAPPLE

1 banana
2 spears of pineapple
3 tbsp low-fat yogurt

Peel the banana and break into slices. Remove the pineapple skin and cut into spears, then chunks. Put all the ingredients into the blender and blend until smooth.

BANANA AND PEACH WITH BERRIES

1 banana
2 peaches
12 strawberries, raspberries or blueberries
3 tbsp low-fat yogurt

Peel and cut the banana. Remove stones from the peaches and cut into chunks. Remove the green stalks from the strawberries. Put all the ingredients into the blender and blend until smooth.

TOFU SHAKE

4 oz/115 g/½ cup tofu
5 oz/140 g fresh or frozen fruit, according to taste
4 fl oz/120 ml/½ cup water
4 fl oz/120 ml/½ cup soy milk
1 tbsp flaxseed oil
9 toasted almonds
4–6 ice cubes (optional)
Sesame seeds

Combine all the ingredients in a blender and mix until smooth and
creamy. Pour into a large glass, sprinkle with sesame seeds and serve cold.

FRESH FRUITS

6-oz/170 g container low-fat fruit yogurt
5 oz/140 g 'matching' fruit – if you used orange yogurt, add fresh or
Frozen oranges
4 fl oz/120 ml/½ cup calcium-enriched non-fat milk

Throw all into a blender and blend.

BLUEBERRY SMOOTHIE

8 oz/230 g blueberry yogurt
5 oz/140 g/1 cup sliced strawberries
8 fl oz/240 ml/1 cup non-fat milk
6 ice cubes

Put all ingredients in a blender and blend.

SALADS

POTATO AND VEGETABLE SALAD

   10 new potatoes with skins on
   Black pepper and sea salt
   2 tbsp cold-pressed olive oil
   4 oz/115 g/2 cups broccoli
   18 oz/510 g/6 cups washed lettuce, torn into small pieces
   4 oz/115 g/2 cups chopped spinach
   3 oz/85 g/1 cup alfalfa sprouts
   2 oz/55 g/1 cup sliced red cabbage
   4 oz/115 g/½ cup low-fat mayonnaise

Boil the potatoes for approximately 20 minutes until tender. Drain, cool
and cut them into chunks. Put in a bowl and add the pepper, salt and oil;
toss well. Place potato mixture on greaseproof paper and bake at
190°C/375°F/Gas Mark 5 for 10 minutes.

Steam the broccoli for a few minutes until tender. Plunge into cold water
for approximately 1 minute and drain well.

Place lettuce and spinach in a bowl, then add the sprouts and red cabbage.
Cut broccoli lengthwise and add to these greens. Add the mayonnaise.

Remove the potatoes from the oven and add them to the salad.

FRUITY CARROT SALAD* *Serves 2*

   8 oz/230 g/1½ cups carrots
   1 small orange
   2 oz/60 g/scant ½ cup raisins
   1 tbsp freshly grated ginger root

Put washed and grated carrots into a bowl, and segment the orange so that the juice falls onto the carrots. Add the orange segments to the carrots. Add the raisins and ginger and fold the ingredients together. Serve chilled.

MUSHROOM SALAD* *Serves 2*

> 8 oz/230 g/2 cups button mushrooms, sliced
> 1 clove garlic, crushed
> 1 tsp sunflower oil
> Hint of lemon juice
> ½ oz/15 g/¼ cup chopped parsley

Add sliced mushrooms and crushed garlic to a pan and heat in the oil for five minutes. Add the lemon juice and stir for about 1 minute. Pour into a serving dish and chill for 1 hour. Serve sprinkled with the parsley.

PASTA SALAD* *Serves 2*

> 4 oz/115 g/1½ cups wholewheat pasta
> ½ tbsp olive oil
> Half an onion, diced
> half a clove garlic, crushed
> ½ oz/15 g/½ cup basil leaves, chopped
> 2 tbsp tomato purée (paste)

Cook pasta as normal. Heat the oil in a pan. Add the onion and garlic and fry to soften the onion. Stir in the basil and tomato purée (paste).

Mix the pasta with the onion mixture and leave to cool. Serve chilled.

(This is a good salad for between-meals snacks as it can easily be packed into a container and taken with you to work.)

GREEN SALAD *Serves 4*

Lettuce heart and rest of the lettuce
Sliced cucumber (half)
4 spring onions (scallions)
Bunch watercress
1 tbsp olive oil

Dressing
2 tbsp lemon juice
1 teaspoon honey
1 clove garlic, crushed
Pinch black pepper
Pinch mustard powder

Prepare the salad – lettuce, cucumber, spring onions (scallions) and watercress – and put in the fridge. Just before serving, add the olive oil and the dressing.

CHEESE, CUCUMBER, ORANGE AND RED PEPPER SALAD
Serves 4

6 oz/170 g/1½ cup low-fat cheddar cheese, cut into cubes
1 large red (bell) pepper
1 small cucumber, cut into chunks
12 anchovies
Half a small lettuce

Mix the salad ingredients in a bowl and chill. Add a low-fat dressing of your choice before serving. Garnish with the anchovies.

GREEN PEPPER AND SWEETCORN SALAD *Serves 4*

8 oz/230 g/2⅔ cups French (green) beans
6 oz/170 g tin sweetcorn
2 spring onions (scallions), thinly sliced
2 tbsp low-fat French dressing

Cook the beans in slightly salted water until tender. Drain, refresh in cold, running water and leave to cool. Mix the beans, sweetcorn and onions (scallions) and stir together with the French dressing.

GREEK SALAD *Serves 2*

1 large tomato, cut into segments
¼ onion, sliced fine
¼ green or red (bell) pepper, sliced fine
Cucumber pieces, peeled and sliced – as much as desired
4-6 black olives
2 oz/60 g/1 cup feta cheese
3 tbsp olive oil
Pinch of salt and dried oregano

Mix all the ingredients in a bowl and serve.

MEXICAN BEAN SALAD

Half an 8-oz/230-g tin black beans, drained
4 oz/115 g/½ cup tinned sweetcorn, drained
Low-fat dressing of your choice
6 oz/170 g/2 cups leaf lettuce, washed, dried and torn into small pieces
1 fresh tomato, chopped
1 oz/30 g/¼ cup cheddar cheese, grated

Mix the beans and sweetcorn with the dressing and leave for an hour or

so. Put washed lettuce on two plates and spoon over the bean mixture.
Add the tomatoes and sprinkle cheese on top.

TUNA SALAD WITH SOY NUTS *Serves 2*

8 oz/230 g/1⅓ cups water-packed tuna
6 oz/170 g/1 cup shredded carrots
1 oz/30 g/¼ cup red onion
4 oz/115 g/⅔ cup feta or goat's cheese
2½ oz/70 g soy nuts
2 oz/60 g/1 cup breadcrumbs

Dressing
2 fl oz/60 ml/¼ cup olive oil
2 tbsp lemon juice
Pinch black pepper
1 clove garlic, crushed

Put the salad ingredients in a bowl. Mix the dressing ingredients
separately. Toss the salad with the dressing and serve.

SPINACH WITH TOFU SALAD

6 oz/170 g/¾ cup tofu
4 tbsp lemon juice (for the tofu)
1 tbsp powdered ginger
1 tsp black pepper
4 oz/115 g/2 cups fresh spinach
2½ oz/70 g/½ cup sliced carrots
2 oz/60 g/½ cup sliced green (bell) pepper
1 tsp soy sauce
1 tbsp white vinegar
1 tbsp water
1 tbsp olive oil

1 garlic clove, crushed
Juice from quarter of a lemon (for the salad dressing)

Cut the tofu into chunks and add the lemon juice, ginger and pepper. Put on a lightly greased baking tray and cook until brown. Combine the spinach, carrots and green (bell) pepper. Mix together the soy sauce, white vinegar, water, olive oil, garlic and lemon and pour this dressing over the salad. Add the tofu and toss well. Serve with a slice of wholewheat toast.

CHICKEN AND TARRAGON SALAD* *Serves 2*

2½ fl oz/70 ml/¼ cup low-fat mayonnaise
2½ fl oz/70 ml/¼ cup low-fat yogurt
1 tbsp freshly chopped tarragon
6 oz/170 g/1¼ cups cooked chicken (skin removed) or tofu, cut into strips

Mix the mayonnaise, yogurt and tarragon together in a large bowl; gently fold into the chicken or tofu. Chill and serve with a large, mixed salad.

SOUPS

PEA AND MUSHROOM SOUP

1 tbsp olive oil
1 onion, chopped
2 cloves garlic, peeled and chopped
1 carrot, chopped
3 oz/85 g/¾ cup mushrooms
32 fl oz/960 ml/4 cups water or chicken broth
6 oz/170 g/¾ cup split green peas
Pinch of black pepper and salt to taste

In a large pan, sauté the onion, garlic, carrot and mushrooms until soft.

Add water or chicken broth and peas. Reduce heat and simmer for 45 minutes or until peas are soft.

LENTIL SOUP* *Serves 2*

4 oz/115 g/2 cups red lentils
12 fl oz/425 ml/1½ cups vegetable stock
4 fl oz/120 ml/½ cup water
Half an onion
1 clove garlic
½ tsp sunflower oil
Pinch ground cumin
2 wedges lemon

Pour the lentils into a pan, add the stock and water and bring to boiling point. Simmer for 30 minutes and remove any scum that rises to the surface with a wooden spoon. Peel and chop the onion. Peel and crush the garlic. Heat the oil in a non-stick frying pan over a moderate heat. Fry the onion and garlic until brown. Add the cumin to the lentils and stir well. Serve the soup in indvidual bowls and garnish with the onion/garlic mixture and lemon. Served with wholemeal bread, this is a nutritious and tasty snack.

BROCCOLI SOUP *Serves 6*

8 oz/230 g/4 cups broccoli, chopped
40 fl oz/1½ litres/5 cups vegetable stock
Pinch salt
2 tbsp non-fat milk
Pinch nutmeg and cayenne or black pepper

Put the broccoli, stock and salt in a large saucepan, bring to the boil, reduce heat and simmer for 20 minutes. Remove from the heat and blend the mixture to a puree with the milk, nutmeg and cayenne. Return to pan, heat through, do not boil.

VEGETABLE SOUP *Serves 4*

4 tbsp extra virgin olive oil
1 large onion, chopped fine
2 cloves garlic, chopped fine
2 large courgettes (zucchini), trimmed and grated
4 new potatoes, scrubbed and grated
1 large carrot, grated
Vegetables of your choice (for example 1 lb/500 g/4½ cups Brussels
sprouts, 2 stalks celery, 3 large leeks, a tin of peas. Or you might prefer to
add a tin of soybeans or flageolet beans)
52 fl oz/1.5 litres/5¼ cups vegetable stock

Heat the oil. Add the onion and garlic and sweat gently for 5 minutes. Add
the grated and chopped vegetables and heat for 5 more minutes, stirring
all the time. Put the stock in and let it simmer for 10 minutes. Remove
from the pan, blend until smooth, then return to pan. Rinse the beans and
peas if you want to include them. Add to the pan, bring back to a simmer
and heat for 5 minutes.

COUSCOUS SOUP

1 small onion, chopped
2 large tomatoes, chopped
2 cloves garlic, chopped
1 8-fl oz/240-ml tin vegetable broth
6 oz/170 g/1 cup precooked (according to instructions on packet) couscous
Salt and pepper to taste

Sauté the onion, tomatoes and garlic in small amount of olive oil. Add the
broth and couscous. Bring to boiling point, but don't boil. Season and
serve with Parmesan cheese according to taste.

HARICOT (NAVY) BEAN SOUP *Serves 5*

7 oz/200 g/1 cup haricot (navy) beans, picked clean and soaked overnight
1 medium onion, sliced thin
2 carrots, sliced thin
2 small celery sticks, sliced thin
14 oz/400 g/1¾ cups chopped tomatoes
1 teaspoon tomato purée (paste)
4½ fl oz/150 ml/⅔ cup olive oil
2 tbsp fresh parsley, chopped
Sea salt and black pepper

Wash and drain the beans. Cover with water in a pan and boil for 3–5 minutes, drain again and discard the water. Return the beans to the pan with 850ml/1½ pints/3¾ cups of water and add the rest of the ingredients apart from the parsley and seasonings. Cover and cook for about 1 hour or until the beans are soft. Add the salt, pepper and parsley and simmer for about 5 minutes before serving.

BROCCOLI AND CHEESE SOUP *Serves 5*

16 fl oz/480 ml/2 cups low-sodium broth
1 oz/30 g/¼ cup chopped onion
5 oz/140 g dry non-fat milk powder mixed with 4 fl oz/120 ml/½ cup water
½ oz/15 g/¼ cup wholwheat breadcrumbs
4 oz/115 g/1 cup cheddar cheese, shredded
Pinch of black pepper
10 oz/285 g/5 cups chopped broccoli

In a saucepan, heat the broth and onion. Bring to a boil, reduce heat and simmer for 10 minutes. Add the milk to the broth. Bring to a boil, reduce heat and simmer for 10 minutes. Mix remaining water with breadcrumbs, add to the broth, and stir until the soup mixture thickens. Add the cheese, pepper and broccoli; stir and heat until the broccoli is soft.

CARROT SOUP* *Serves 4*

1 lb/455 g/3¼ cups carrots
1 small onion
1 tsp sunflower oil
28 fl oz/850 ml/3¾ cups vegetable stock
1 orange
1 tbsp chopped coriander (cilantro)

Rinse, peel and chop the carrots and the onion. Heat the oil in a pan, add
the onion and fry in a gentle heat for a few minutes. Add the carrots and
cook for around 2 minutes. Add the stock, zest and juice of the orange,
and the coriander (cilantro). Bring to the boil and leave to simmer with the
lid on for about 45 minutes. Put the soup into a blender or food processor
and process till smooth. Rinse the pan. Return the soup to the pan and
heat until very hot. Serve with croutons if desired.

MAIN MEALS

BAKED POTATO

Before cooking your potato, make sure it is washed and scrubbed and
poke it with a fork several times all over to prevent explosion in the oven.
Bake at 180°C/350°F/Gas Mark 4 for about 1 hour.

A great alternative to your basic baked potato is to slice one or two large
potatoes into bite-sized chunks. Spread them on a baking sheet and toss
with a small amount of olive or canola oil. Bake at 190°C/375°F/Gas Mark 5
for about half an hour or until the potato chunks are soft in the middle.

BROWN RICE

Brown rice is much better for you than white rice. You need 16–24 fl oz/450–700ml/2–¾ cups of water for every 8 oz/225 g/1 cup of short or long grain brown rice. Put the water and the rice in a pan and bring to a boil for about a minute. Reduce heat, cover the pan and simmer for about 30 minutes, stirring occasionally, until the rice is tender and the water has gone.

SPANISH OMELETTE *Serves 1*

- **1 small onion, chopped**
- **2 fl oz/60 ml¼ cup water**
- **1 stick celery, chopped**
- **1 green (bell) pepper, chopped**
- **2 eggs**
- **1 tsp butter**
- **2 tomatoes, chopped**

Put the onions and water in a sealed pan over a medium heat. When the water begins to boil, reduce the heat to low. Add the celery and green pepper and cook until soft. Beat the eggs and melt the butter in a frying pan over a low heat. Pour in the beaten eggs and cook gently. Strain the vegetables and tip onto the partly-cooked omelette; add the tomatoes. Serve with a salad.

TUNA (OR SALMON) FISHCAKES*

- **6 oz/170 g/1 cup tinned salmon or tuna**
- **9 oz/260 g/1½ cups mashed potato**
- **1 oz/30 g/½ cup parsley**
- **2 eggs, lightly beaten**
- **1 tbsp wholewheat flour**
- **2 oz/60 g dried wholewheat breadcrumbs**
- **1 tbsp sunflower oil**

Add the salmon to your mashed potato. Add the parsely and half the beaten egg, and fold the mixture together.

Sprinkle the flour on a worksurface and roll the fish mixture into a sausage shape. Cut into 6 or 8 cakes and shape. Dip each in the remaining egg. Then coat with the dried breadcrumbs.

Heat the oil in a non-stick frying pan (skillet). Cook the fishcakes over a moderate heat for a few minutes each side. Drain thoroughly on paper towel. Serve hot with a selection of freshly cooked vegetables, or cold with a large mixed salad.

SALMON DINNER *Serves 1*

> 4 fl oz/120 ml/½ cup non-fat milk
> 4 oz/115 g/⅔ cup salmon
> 1 lemon wedge
> 3 oz/85 g/1 cup steamed broccoli
> 1 clove garlic, chopped
> 1 tbsp flaxseed oil

Heat the non-fat milk in a frying pan (skillet) and add the salmon. Poach the salmon on high heat for 6 or 7 minutes. Check the middle of the fish to see that it is done. Sprinkle with fresh lemon juice. Put the broccoli in a steamer with the garlic and steam for 10 minutes. Top with flaxseed oil. Serve the salmon and broccoli with new potatoes or a baked potato with non-fat sour cream.

RISOTTO *Serves 2–4*

> 1 tbsp olive oil
> 1 medium onion, chopped fine
> Your choice of content: seafood, chicken or veg: mushrooms, asparagus, broad (fava) beans. For veg or chicken add basil or nutmeg; for seafood try lemon juice or thyme.

9 oz/250 g/1¼ cups risotto rice
1 tbsp tomato purée (paste)
20 fl oz/575 ml/2½ cups stock
1 oz/30 g/¼ cup grated low-fat cheese
Parmesan cheese if desired

Gently heat the oil in a pan and add onions and spices. Cook for about 5 minutes, then add your choice of ingredients in order of the amount of time they will take to cook – i.e. if you are using raw chicken, add that first until it is browned, then add the veg. Give it a stir, then add the risotto rice. Add the tomato purée (paste) and stir well before adding the stock. Bring to the boil, then cover and turn down the heat as low as it will go and leave for 15 mins. This should be enough time to cook the rice; if not, add some water. Stir and add the cheese. Allow to stand and cool for a few minutes, sprinkle with Parmesan cheese if you like and serve.

LENTIL CHILLI *Serves 2*

8 oz/230 g/1 heaping cup lentils
40 fl oz/1.2 litres/5 cups water
8 oz/230 g lean pork or turkey or soy beans
1 large onion, chopped
1 clove garlic, peeled and minced
Salt to taste
16 fl oz/480 ml/2 cups tomato sauce
10 fl oz/300 ml/1⅓ cups tomato juice
8 fl oz/240 ml/1 cup cold water
1 tbsp chilli powder

Rinse the lentils and put in a large covered pan with the water. Bring to the boil, reduce heat and simmer for 30 minutes. Drain. Brown your meat or soy beans with the onion, garlic and salt; add to the drained lentils. Add tomato sauce, juice, cold water and chilli powder. Cook for 1 hour over a very low heat to blend all the flavours.

NUT ROAST *Serves 4–6*

1 medium onion
1 oz/30 g/⅛ cup margarine
10 oz/280 g/2 cups mixed nuts
10 fl oz/300 ml/1⅓ cups vegetable stock
2 tsp yeast extract
1 tsp mixed herbs
12 oz/340 g/2 cups cooked brown rice

Chop the onion and sauté in the margarine. Grind the nuts in a blender or food processer. Heat the stock and yeast extract to boiling point, then combine all the ingredients, including the cooked brown rice, and mix well until the mixture is of slack consistency. Turn into a greased shallow baking dish, level the surface and bake at 180°C/350°F/Gas Mark 4 for about 30–35 minutes or until golden brown.

VEGETABLE STEW *Serves 2–6*

1 large onion, chopped
1 large clove garlic, peeled and chopped
1 tbsp olive oil
6 oz/170 g/3 cups fresh spinach, chopped
1 14-oz/400-g tin chickpeas (garbanzo beans)
1 14-oz/400-g large tin tomatoes, chopped
4 or 5 fresh tomatoes, chopped
2½ oz/70 g/½ cup raisins
2 new potatoes, peeled and chopped
3 oz/85 g/scant ½ cup brown rice
Black pepper and salt to taste

Fry the onion and garlic in the olive oil. Add the spinach and cook until limp, then add the rest of the ingredients, except the salt. Cook for 45 minutes or until the potatoes are soft when pricked by a fork. You may need to add a little water if the stew gets too thick. Add the salt and serve.

BROCCOLI, BEANS AND BAKED POTATO DINNER

4 oz/115 g/½ cup cottage cheese
1 tbsp flaxseed oil
Large baked potato
4 oz/115 g/scant ½ cup baked beans
3 oz/85 g/1 cup cut and steamed broccoli

Add the cottage cheese and flaxseed oil to the baked potato and serve with the baked beans and steamed broccoli.

PASTA WITH PESTO AND OIL-RICH FISH

9 oz/260 g/3 cups wheat-free pasta such as corn and vegetable pasta shells
4 oz/115 g pesto sauce (see page 330)
6 oz/170 g/1 cup fresh tuna or salmon (tinning reduces tuna's Omega-3 content)

Cook the pasta in boiling water according to the instructions on the packet. When the pasta is ready, drain and transfer to a warmed serving dish. Add approximately 1 tablespoon of pesto sauce per person and gently mix in with the pasta. Remove any bones from the fish and flake with a fork. Add to the pasta and pesto and mix together.

POTATO OMELETTE*

1 egg
2 oz/60 g/⅓ cup mashed potato
2 spring onions (scallions)
Pinch black pepper
2 tsp sunflower oil

Add the egg to the potato in a mixing bowl and stir well. Chop the onions (scallions) and add these with the pepper to the potato and egg. Stir well.

Heat 1 teaspoon of the oil in a pan, spread the potato mixture in the pan and cook over a low heat for 5 minutes. Place a flat plate over the top of the pan, invert the pan so the omelette falls neatly onto the plate. Put the rest of the oil in the pan and slide the omelette back in. Cook for 5 more minutes, then serve.

VEGETABLE AND CHEESE BAKE* *Serves 4*

1 tbsp sunflower oil
1 small onion, peeled and diced
4 oz/115 g/1⅓ cups mushrooms, chopped
1 small red (bell) pepper, washed, de-seeded and chopped
1 stick celery, washed and chopped
4 oz/115 g/2 cups wholewheat breadcrumbs
2–3 oz/60–90 g/½–¾ cup grated low-fat hard cheese
1 egg, lightly beaten

Heat the oil in a frying pan (skillet), add the onion and fry for a few minutes. Add the mushrooms, pepper and celery and cook for a few more minutes. Turn the heat down and add the breadcrumbs, cheese and egg. Mix well. Pour the mixture into a lightly greased loaf tin and bake at 190°C/375°F/Gas Mark 5 for about an hour. Remove from the oven and let stand for 15 minutes. Serve with jacket potato, salad or fresh vegetables and tomato sauce.

TOFU AND MUSHROOM KEBABS *Serves 4*

2 tbsp soy sauce
2 tbsp smooth peanut butter
1 tbsp chilli sauce
8 oz/230 g/1 cup tofu, cubed
4 oz/115 g/1 cup button mushrooms

Mix the soy sauce, peanut butter and chilli in a bowl. Add the tofu and mushrooms and stir gently. Leave to stand for 1 hour. Put the tofu and mushrooms on a skewer and grill (broil) for about 2 minutes on each side. Serve hot with rice or salad.

LASAGNA WITH BEANS

1 tsp garlic, chopped
1 small onion, chopped
1 tbsp canola oil
12 oz/340 g/2 cups kidney beans, chopped
16 fl oz/480 ml/2 cups tomato sauce
16 fl oz/480 ml/2 cups tomato purée (paste)
1 tsp basil
8 oz/230 g/1 cup soft tofu
8 oz/230 g/1 cup cottage cheese
12 oz/340 g uncooked lasagna noodles
6 oz/170 g/1 cup mozzarella cheese

Sauté the garlic and onion in the oil. Stir in the beans. Add tomato sauce, puree (paste) and basil to taste. Bring to the boil, reduce heat and simmer for 10 minutes.

Mix the tofu with the cottage cheese.

Spread a little of the bean mixture on the bottom of a 9-inch glass baking dish. Layer a third of the noodles on top of the beans. On top of the noodles put half your cottage cheese-tofu mixture. Then add the mozzarella. Keep repeating layers until everything is used up. Cover with foil and bake for about an hour at 190°C/375°F/Gas Mark 5 or until the noodles are soft.

DAHL

9 oz/250 g/1¼ cups red lentils
20 fl oz/575 ml/2½ cups water
½ tsp cumin
½ tsp coriander (cilantro)
1 tsp olive oil
1 tbsp black mustard seeds
1 small onion, chopped
Salt and pepper to taste
Splash of milk

Put the lentils in a pan. Cover with the water, add the spices and bring to the boil, then reduce heat. Simmer until the lentils have absorbed all the water and are soft. Once these are cooked, put them to one side.

Gently heat the oil and add the mustard seeds. Once most of the seeds have popped, add the onion and stir until really soft. Then add the lentil mixture and seasoning and stir well. Add milk to loosen the mixture a little.

PESTO* *Serves 2–3*

1 oz/30 g/1 cup fresh basil leaves
1 tbsp roasted pine nuts
1 clove garlic, crushed
1 fl oz/30 ml/2 tbsp sunflower oil
½ oz/15 g/¼ cup Parmesan cheese, grated
8 oz/230 g fresh wholewheat pasta

Put the basil, pine nuts, garlic and oil into a blender and process to get a smooth taste. Pour into a bowl and add the cheese. Cook the pasta according to the instructions on the packet. Drain thoroughly. Serve the pesto with piping hot pasta and cheese. This dish goes well with a mixed side salad and wholewheat bread rolls to mop up the sauce.

EGG AND SPINACH CAKE* *Serves 4*

4 oz/115 g/½ cup risotto rice
½ tsp sunflower oil
1 small onion
4 oz/115 g/2 cups frozen spinach
2 eggs
2 oz/60 g/1 cup freshly grated Parmesan cheese
Pinch black pepper

Cook the risotto rice according to the instructions on the packet. Put the oil in a pan, add the onion and fry until the onion is light brown. Put the frozen spinach, risotto and onion in a bowl. Crack the eggs and lightly beat the whites and yokes together. Add the eggs, cheese, and pepper to the spinach, risotto and onion mixture and stir thoroughly. Transfer to a cake tin and bake for about 30 minutes in a hot oven (approximately 200°C/400°F/Gas Mark 6).

DESSERTS

DRIED FRUIT COMPOTE* *Serves 2*

1 oz/30 g/⅙ cup dried figs
1 oz/30 g/⅓ cup dried apricots
1 oz/30 g/⅓ cup dried prunes
1 oz/30 g/⅓ cup dried apple
1 oz/30 g/⅙ cup raisins
4 fl oz/120 ml/½ cup apple juice

Put the dried fruits into a bowl with the apple juice and leave in the fridge overnight. Serve chilled.

BAKED APPLE WITH STUFFING

    2 good-sized cooking apples
    1 tbsp honey or sugar-free jam
    Stuffing suggestions: dates, cinnamon, raisins

Core the apples and slit skins in a ring round the middle. Stuff with your chosen filling and the honey. Bake until fruit is tender. Serve hot or cold.

FRUIT KEBABS

If you don't find fruit all that appealing, here's a way to make it more interesting. Buy a pack of wooden skewers from your supermarket. Cut your fruit into 1-inch squares and thread on your skewers. Try alternating chunks of pineapple with melon, peach, apricots, bananas and grapes.

BANANA SURPRISE* *Serves 3*

    2 bananas
    1 oz/30 g/⅕ cup dates, chopped
    1 oz/30 g/⅐ cup dried apricots, chopped
    1 oz/30 g/⅙ cup seedless grapes, chopped
    1 oz/30 g/¼ cup almonds, chopped

Mash the bananas in a bowl and stir in the dates, apricots, grapes and nuts. Spread the mixture in a freezer tray and freeze for 2 hours. Serve chilled.

FRUIT AND OATCAKE DESSERT

    2 bananas
    2 apples
    8 dried apricots

Water as needed
8–12 oatcakes
2 oz/60 g/½ cup broken walnuts

Peel, rinse, remove pips and cut all the fruit into small pieces and put into
a saucepan. Add a few tablespoons of water and simmer for 10 minutes or
until the fruit is soft, adding more water if the mixture becomes too dry.
Put the oakcakes into the bottom of your dessert bowls – you may have to
break the oatcakes to make them fit. When the fruit is soft, pour over the
oatcakes. Serve with a sprinkling of walnuts.

BRULÉE

Fruit of your choice
8 oz/230 g/1 cup low-fat fromage frais or Greek-style yogurt
Demerara sugar

Line the bottom of a ramekin with your fruit, then add the yogurt to fill to
the top and sprinkle with sugar. Place under a pre-heated grill (broiler)
until the sugar starts to bubble.

FRUIT AND NUT SALAD *Serves 4*

1 peach, sliced
2 oranges, sliced
8 oz/230 g/1 heaping cup fresh pineapple, chopped
6 oz/170 g/1 cup seedless grapes, chopped
1 oz/30 g/⅕ cup Brazil nuts, chopped
Juice of 1 orange
Handful of toasted almonds

Put peach slices and orange slices into four serving bowls. Mix the
pineapple, grapes and nuts and place on top of the peach and orange
slices. Spoon over the orange juice and sprinkle with toasted almonds.

FRUIT LOAF

11 oz/300 g/2 heaping cups wholewheat flour
1 tbsp baking powder
6 oz/175 g/1 scant cup muscovado sugar
1 egg
1 medium banana – mashed
8 oz/230 g/1 cup low-fat Greek yogurt
Handful of raisins

Add the wholewheat flour and baking powder to a bowl and stir in the sugar. Add the rest of the ingredients and spoon into a greased loaf tin. Heat at 180°C/350°F/Gas Mark 4 for about 40 minutes. Make sure the centre is well cooked before you remove from the oven.

RAISIN AND PUMPKIN BREAD PUDDING

20 oz/570 g/10 cups pumpkin purée (paste)
4 fl oz/120 ml/½ cup honey
4 fl oz/120 ml/½ cup melted butter
2 eggs
4 fl oz/120 ml/½ cup milk
2½ oz/70 g/½ cup raisins
2 oz/60 g/½ cup walnuts, chopped
1½ oz/45 g/½ cup rolled oats
5 oz/145 g/1 cup wholewheat flour
1 tbsp baking powder
½ tsp ground cinnamon
¼ tsp ground nutmeg
¼ tsp ground ginger
¼ tsp ground cloves
Pinch salt

Mix the pumpkin, honey, melted butter and eggs in a bowl. Stir in milk, raisins and walnuts.

In another bowl, mix the dry ingredients and make a big well in the centre. Pour in the pumpkin and raisin mixture and blend the ingredients. Pour into a well-greased loaf pan and bake in a preheated oven (180°C/350°F/Gas Mark 4) for 1 hour. Let cool for half an hour before cutting.

YOGURT PUDDING* *Serves 2*

   2 bananas
   4 fl oz/120 ml/½ cup soy yogurt
   1 tsp vanilla essence (extract)
   1 oz/30 g/¼ cup toasted almonds

Mash the bananas in a large bowl. Add the yogurt and vanilla essence (extract) and stir well. Put the mixture into a tin and freeze for 2 hours. Serve in individual dishes and sprinke with toasted almonds.

RICE PUDDING *Serves 2*

   2 oz/60 g pudding rice
   1 tbsp caster sugar
   10 fl oz/300 ml/1⅓ cups non-fat milk
   1 tbsp vanilla essence (extract)
   2 tbsp low-sugar raspberry jam

Put the rice, sugar and milk in a pan and cook on a low heat until the mixture starts to bubble. Leave to simmer for 15 minutes. Stir in the vanilla essence (extract). Spoon into serving dishes. Serve hot or cold with a spoonful of low-sugar raspberry jam.

RED FRUIT DESSERT* *Serves 2*

4 oz/115 g/⅔ cup strawberries
4 oz/115 g/1 cup raspberries
2 oz/60 g/⅓ cup redcurrants
2 fl oz/60 ml/¼ cup unsweetened cranberry or apple juice

Remove leaves and stems and wash the fruit under cold, running water. Put the fruit into a bowl and stir in the cranberry or apple juice. Chill for half an hour and serve with low-fat yogurt or low-fat vanilla ice-cream.

APPLE CRUNCH *Serves 4*

1 lb/455 g/4 cups cooking apples, sliced
2 tbsp lemon juice
2 tbsp water
2 oz/60 g/¼ cup margarine
1 oz/30 g/⅙ cup brown sugar
2 oz/60 g/½ cup almonds
4 oz/115 g/2 cups wholewheat breadcrumbs

Put the apples into a pan with the lemon juice and water. Cook for 10 minutes on a moderate heat. Melt the margarine in a frying pan (skillet) over a low heat. Add the brown sugar, almonds and breadcrumbs. Stir well. Put the lightly stewed apple into a pie dish and top with the breadcrumb mixture. Bake at 180°C/350°F/Gas Mark 4 for 30 to 40 minutes. Serve hot or cold.

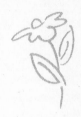

Suggested Reading

Acne/Skincare
Good Skin Doctor, Anne Lovell, Tony Chu (Thorsons)
Natural Beauty: Natural Approaches to Skin and Hair Care, Sidra Shaukat
    (Health Essentials)

Additives
E is for Additives, Maurice Hanssen, Jill Marsden (Thorsons)
How to Avoid GM food, Joanna Blythman (Fourth Estate)

Alternative Therapies
Alternative Medicine for Dummies, James Dillard and Terra Ziporyn
    (Dummies press/IDG books)
Alternative Therapy – The Definitive Guide, Burton Goldberg (Future Medicine
    Publishing Inc)
The Hamlyn Encyclopedia of Complementary Therapies (Hamlyn)
Women's Encyclopedia of Natural Medicine, Tori Hudson (McGraw Hill)

Cookbooks
Cooking Without, Barbara Cousins (Thorsons)
Erica White's Beat Candida Cookbook (Thorsons)

The Good Carb Cookbook: Secrets of Eating Low on the GI, Sandra Woodruff
(Avery)
Gourmet Prescription, Deborah Friedson Chud (Bay Books)
The Optimum Nutrition Cookbook, Patrick Holford (Piatkus)
PMS: Over 100 Recipes for Overcoming PMS, Jill Davies (Thorsons)
PMS: Recipes for Health, Jill Davies (Thorsons)
The Sunday Times Vitality Cookbook, Susan Clarke (HarperCollins)
Vegetarian Cooking Without, Barbara Cousins (Thorsons)

Depression
Burned Out and Blue, Kristina Dowling Orr (Thorsons)
Overcoming Depression: What therapy doesn't teach you and can't give you,
Richard O'Conner (Berkley Publishing Group)
St John's Wort: Your Natural Prozac, Norman Rosenthal (Thorsons)

Diet/Nutrition
Beat Sugar Craving: The revolutionary four-week diet, Maryon Stewart
(Vermillion)
Body Foods for Women, Jane Clarke (Orion)
Foods That Harm, Foods That Heal (Reader's Digest)
Glucose Revolution: Guide to the Glycemic Index, Thomas Wolever (Marlowe)
Healing with Whole Foods, Paul Pitchford (North Atlantic)
Prescription for Nutritional Healing, James and Phyllis Balch (Avery)
Sugar Busters, H. Leighton Stewart (Ballantine)

Endometriosis
Endometriosis: A key to healing through nutrition, Dian Shepperson Mills and
Michael Vernon (Thorsons)

Fatigue
The Beat Fatigue Handbook, Erica White (Thorsons)

Fitness books/videos
Be Your Best, Sally Gunnell (Thorsons)
Complete Book of Yoga, Vimla Lalvani (Hamlyn)
The Complete Illustrated Guide to Yoga, Howard Kent (Element)

Diets Don't Work, Vimla Lalvani, Lace International VHS
The Idiot's Guide to Fitness, Claire Walker (Alpha)
Introduction to Tai Chi, Lucy Lloyd-Barker, Inc Vision Ltd, VHS
Rosemary Conley fitness videos, BBC Worldwide and Video Collection Inc,
    VHS

Food and Mood
Emotional Health, Deborah Sichel (William Morrow)
Food and Mood, Elizabeth Somer (Owl Books)
The Food and Mood Handbook, Amanda Geary (Thorsons)
Women's Moods: What Every Woman Should Know about Hormones, the Brain
    and Emotional Health, Deborah Sichel, Jean Watson Driscoll
    (HarperCollins)

Giving Up Smoking
Allen Carr's Easy Way to Stop Smoking (Penguin)
Breathe Easy: The Friendly Stop-Smoking Guide for Women, Susannah Hayward
    (Penguin)
Stop Smoking Naturally, Martha Work (Keats)

Herbal Medicine
The Complete Woman's Herbal, Anne McIntyre (Henry Holt)
Herbal Defence, Robyn Landis (Thorsons)
Herbal Remedies for Women, Amanda Crawford (Prima)
Holistic Woman's Herbal, Kitty Campion (Bloomsbury)

Hormones
Androgen Disorders in Women: The Most Neglected Hormone Problem, Theresa
    Francis Cheung and James Douglas (Hunter House)
Balancing Hormones Naturally, Kate Neil and Patrick Holford (Piatkus)
The Good News about Women's Hormones, Geoffrey Redmond (Warner)

Natural/Well Woman
Complete Women's Health (Royal College of Obstetricians and
    Gynaecologists)
The Natural Health Handbook for Women, Marilyn Glenville (Piatkus)

Our Bodies Our Selves for the New Century, Boston Women's Health Collective (Touchstone)
Women's Bodies, Women's Wisdom, Christine Northrup (Bantam)
Women's Encyclopedia of Natural Medicine, Tori Hudson (McGraw Hill)

Organic Living

Organic Living: Simple Solutions for a Better Life, Lynda Brown (DK Publishing)
Organic Living in 10 Simple Lessons, Karen Sullivan (Barnes Ed)
Taste Life: The Organic Choice, David Richard, (Vital Health)

PCOS

The PCOS Diet Book, Colette Harris, Theresa Cheung (Thorsons)

Perimenopause

Before the Change: Taking charge of your perimenopause, Ann Louise Gittleman (HarperSanFrancisco)

PMS

PMS: The Essential Guide to Treatment Options, Katharina Dalton and David Holton (Thorsons)

Self-esteem

Self-esteem, Gael Lindenfield (Thorsons)
Self-esteem Companion, Matthew McKay (New Harbinger)
611 Ways to Boost Your Self-esteem, Bryan Robinson (Health Communications)
10 Days to Great Self-esteem, David Burns (Vermillion)

Stress

The Little Book of Calm, Paul Wilson (Penguin)
101 Shortcuts to Relaxation, Cathy Hopkins (Bloomsbury)
Stress, Anxiety and Insomnia, Michael Murray (Prima)
Stressbusters, Robert Holden (Thorsons)
Write Your Own Prescription for Stress, Kenneth Matheny (New Harbinger)

Supplements

Earl Mindell's Supplement Bible (Thorsons)
The Nutritional Health Bible, Linda Lazarides (Thorsons)
The Optimum Nutrition Bible, Patrick Holford, Piatkus
Reader's Digest Guide to Vitamins, Minerals and Supplements
Thorsons Complete Guide to Vitamins and Minerals, Leonard Mervyn
    (Thorsons)

Thyroid

Thyroid Problems, Patsy Westcott (Thorsons)
Thyroid – Why Am I So Tired?, Martin Budd (Thorsons)

Weight Loss

Lighten Up, Pete Cohen, Judith Verity (Century)
The Zone: A Dietary Road Map to Lose Weight Permanently, Barry Sears
    (HarperCollins)

References

Part One

Why You Need to Deal with PMS

1 Reid, Robert L., M.D., and Yen, S. S. C., M.D., *American Journal of Obstetrics and Gynecology*, 1981, vol. 139, no. 85, 97

2 DeGraff Bender, Stephanie and Kelleher, Kathleen, *PMS: Women Tell Women How to Control Premenstrual Syndrome* (New Harbinger Publications, 1996) p. 131

3 Dalton, Katharina, M.D., *The Premenstrual Syndrome and Progesterone Therapy* (2nd edition, Year Book Medical Publishers, Inc., 1984), p. viii; Rubinow, David R., M.D. and Roy-Byrne, Peter, M.D., 'Premenstrual Syndromes: Overview from a Methodological Perspective', *American Journal of Psychiatry*, 1984, vol. 141, no. 2, 163

4 Halbreich, U., 'Menstrually Related Disorder: What We Do Know, What We Only Believe That We Know and What We Know That We Do Not Know', *Critical Reviews in Neurobiology*, 1995, vol. 9, 163–74

5 Facchinettie, F. *et al.*, 'Oestradiol/progesterone and the Pre-Menstrual Syndrome', *Lancet*, 1983, vol. 2, 1302; Abraham, G. E., 'Nutritional Factors in the Aetiology of the Pre-menstrual Tension Syndrome', *Journal of Reproductive Medicine*, 1987, vol. 28, 446–64

6 Clare, A., 'Pre-menstrual Syndrome – Single or Multiple Causes', *Canadian Journal of Psychiatry*, 1985, vol. 30, 474–82

7   Eriksson, E. *et al.*, 'Serum Levels of Androgens Are Higher in Women with Pre-menstrual Irritability and Dysphoria Than in Controls', *Psychoneuroimmunology*, 1995, vol. 17, nos 2–3, 195–204

8   Schmidt, P. J. *et al.*, 'Thyroid Function in Women with Pre-menstrual Syndrome', *The Journal of Clinical Endocrinology and Metabolism*, 1993, vol. 76, 671–4

9   Abraham, 'Nutritional Factors in the Aetiology of the Pre-menstrual Tension Syndrome'

10 Thys-Jacob, S., 'Disturbances in Calcium Regulation in Women with PMS', *American Journal of Obstetrics and Gynecology*, August 1998

11 Stewart, A., 'Clinical and Biochemical Effects of Nutritional Supplementation on the Pre-Menstrual Syndrome', *Journal of Reproductive Medicine*, 1987, vol. 32, no. 6, 435–41; Gallant, M. P., 'Pyridoxine and Magnesium Status in Women with Pre-menstrual Syndrome', *Nutrition Research*, 1987, vol. 7, 243–52

12 Abraham, G. E. and Lubran, M. M., 'Serum and Red Cell Magnesium Levels in Patients with Pre-menstrual Tension', *American Journal of Clinical Nutrition*, 1981, vol. 34, 2364–6; Rosenstein, D. L. *et al.*, 'Magnesium Measures Across the Menstrual Cycles in Pre-menstrual Syndrome', *Biological Psychiatry*, 1994, vol. 35, 557–61

13 Clare, A., 'Pre-menstrual Syndrome: Single or Multiple Causes?', *Canadian Journal of Psychiatry*, 1985, vol. 30, 474–82

14 Winenman, E. W., 'Automatic Balance Changes During the Human Menstrual Cycle', *Psychophysiology*, 1971, vol. 8, no. 1, 1–6; Soules, M. R. *et al.*, 'Luteal Phase Deficiency: Characterization of Reproductive Hormones Over the Menstrual Cycle', *Journal of Clinical Endocrine Metabolism*, 1989, vol. 69, 804–12; Zuckerman, S., 'The Menstrual Cycle', *Lancet*, 18 June, 1949

15 Schmidt, P.J. *et al.*, 'Differential Behavioral Effects of Gonadal Steroids in Women With and Without PMS', *New England Journal of Medicine*, 1998, vol. 338, no. 4, 209–16

16 American College of Obstetrics and Gynecology Opinion, 'Pre-menstrual syndrome', *International Journal of Gynecology and Obstetrics*, 1995, vol. 50, 80–4

How and Why the 12-week Plan Works

1   Wurtman, J. J. *et al.*, 'Effect of Nutrient Intake on Pre-menstrual Tension', *American Journal of Obstetrics and Gynaecology*, 1989, vol. 161, no. 5, 1228–34

2   Goei, G. S., 'Dietary Patterns of Patients with Pre-menstrual Tension', *Journal of Applied Nutrition*, 1982, vol. 34, 4–11

3 De Souza, M. C. *et al.*, 'A Synergistic Effect of a Daily Supplement for One Month of 200mg Magnesium and 50mg Vitamin B6 for the Relief of Anxiety Related PMS: A Randomized Double-bind, Crossover Study', *Journal of Women's Health and Gender Based Medicine*, 2000, vol. 9, no. 2, 131–9

4 Dalton, Katharina, M.D., PMS: *The Essential Guide to Treatment Options* (Thorsons, 1994), p. 69

5 Makela, S. I. *et al.*, 'Dietary Soybean May Be Antiestrogenic in Mice', *Journal of Nutrition*, 1997, vol. 125, no. 3, 437–45; Barnard N. D. et al., 'Diet and Sex-hormone Binding Globulin, Dysmenorrhea and Premenstrual Syndrome', *Obstetrics and Gynaecology*, 2000, vol. 95, no. 2, 245–50

6 Johnson, W. G. *et al.*, 'Macronutrient Intake, Eating Habit and Exercise as Moderators of Menstrual Distress in Healthy Women', *Psychosomatic Medicine*, 1995, vol. 57, 324–30

7 Byrne, A. *et al.*, 'The Effect of Exercise on Depression, Anxiety and Other Mood States: A Review', *Journal of Psychosomatic Research*, 1993, vol. 37, 565–74

8 Goodale, I. L., *et al.*, 'Alleviation of PMS Symptoms with the Relaxation Response', *Obstetrics and Gynaecology*, 1990, vol. 75, 649–55; Woods, N. E. et al., 'Major Life Events, Daily Stressors and PMS Symptoms', *Nursing Research*, 1985, vol. 34, 263–7

9 Abraham, G. E. and Rumley, R. E., 'Role of Nutrition in Managing the Premenstrual Tension Syndromes', *Journal of Reproductive Medicine*, June 1987, 32(6), 405-22; Glenville, Marilyn, Ph.D., *The Nutritional Health Handbook for Women* (Piatkus, 2001), p. 99; Stewart, Maryon and Stewart, Dr Alan, *No More PMS* (Vermillion, 1997)

10 Puolakka, J. *et al.*, 'Biochemical and Clinical Effects of Treating the Pre-menstrual Syndrome with Prostaglandin Synthesis Precursors', *Journal of Reproductive Medicine*, 1985, vol. 30, 149–55; Melanby, A., Best, L., Stevens, A., 'Evening Primrose Oil for Cyclical Mastalgia', Development and Evaluation Committee Report No. 65, December 1996, Research and Development Directorate, Wessex Institute for Health Research and Development

11 Graham, J., *Evening Primrose Oil* (Thorsons, 1984), pp. 37–8

Getting to Know Your Own PMS

1 PMS is not always bad. Some women do report positive symptoms, such as increased energy, more creative thoughts than usual and an increased productivity. If this is you, don't worry, following the plan won't stop this happening. You'll still feel energetic and creative but this won't just be for a few days before your period. You'll feel terrific all month long.

2 Oestrogen is not one hormone but the name used for several hormones, including estrogen and oestradiol, which ensure that a woman matures from childhood to womanhood.

Part Two

Week 1

1 Rossignol, A. M., 'Caffeine-containing Beverages and Pre-menstrual Syndrome in Young Women', *American Journal of Public Health*, 1985, 75 (11), 1335–37

2 Rossignol, A. M. and Bonnlander, H., 'Prevalence and Severity of the Pre-menstrual Syndrome: Effects of Foods and Beverages That Are Sweet or High in Sugar Content', *Journal of Reproductive Medicine*, 1991, vol. 36, no. 2, 131–6

3 Abraham and Lubran, 'Serum and Red Cell Magnesium Levels in Patients with Pre-menstrual Tension'

4 De Souza, 'A Synergistic Effect of a Daily Supplement for One Month of 200mg Magnesium and 50mg Vitamin B6 for the Relief of Anxiety Related PMS: A Randomized Double Bind Crossover Study'; Walker, A. F. *et al.*, 'Magnesium Supplementation Alleviates PMS Symptoms of Fluid Retention', *Journal of Women's Health*, 1998, vol. 7, no. 9, 1157–65

5 Speigel, K. *et al.*, 'Impact of Sleep Debt on Metabolic and Endocrine Function', *Lancet*, 1999, vol. 354, 1435–99

Week 2

1 Thys-Jacob, S., 'Calcium Carbonate and the Pre-menstrual Syndrome: Effects on Premenstrual and Menstrual Symptoms', Premenstrual Syndrome Study Group, *American Journal of Obstetrics and Gynaecology*, 1998, vol. 179, no. 2, 444–52

2 Thys-Jacob, S., 'Micronutrients and the Pre-menstrual Syndrome: the Case of Calcium', *Journal of the American College of Nutrition*, 2000, vol. 19, no. 2, 220–7

3 Byrne, A. *et al.*, 'The Effect of Exercise on Depression, Anxiety and Other Mood States: a Review', *Journal of Psychosomatic Research*, 1993, vol. 37, 565–74

4 Brown, J., 'Staying Fit and Staying Well: Physical Fitness as a Moderator of Life Stress', *Journal of Personality and Social Psychology*, 1991, vol. 60, no. 4, 555–61

5 McClouskey, C., 'The Little Finger Test', *Lancet*, December 1973, 1503

6 Hikino, H., *Traditional Remedies and Modern Assessment: the Case of Ginseng* (Medicinal Plant Industry, Wijeskera ROB, CRC Press, 1991), p. 149–66

Week 3

1 Chen, N., 'Individual Differences in Answering the Four Questions for Happiness', Ph.D. diss., University of Georgia, 1996

2 Woods, N. F., *et al.*, 'Major Life Events, Daily Stressors and Perimenstrual Symptoms', *Nursing Research*, 1985, vol. 34, 263–7

3 Goei, 'Dietary Patterns of Patients with PMS'; Rossignol and Bonnlander, 'Prevalence and Severity of the PMS Syndrome: Effects of Foods and Beverages That Are Sweet or High in Sugar Content'

4 Fontaine, K. R., *et al.*, 'Optimism, Social Support and premenstrual Dysphoria', *Journal of Clinical Psychology*, 1997, 53, 243–7; Morse, G., 'Positively Reframing Perceptions of the Menstrual Cycle among Women with Premenstrual Syndrome', *Journal of Obstetrics, Gynecologic and Neonatal Nursing*, 1999, 28, 165–74

5 Thurman, C., 'Personality Correlates of the Type A Behavior Pattern', Ph.D. diss., University of Georgia, 1981

Week 4

1 Lepper, H., 'In Pursuit of Happiness and Satisfaction in Later Life: A Study of Competing Theories of Subjective Wellbeing', Ph.D. diss., University of California, 1996

2 Mokherjee, H., 'Perception of Well-being Among Older Persons in Neometropolitan America', *Perceptual and Motor Skills*, 1997, 85, 943

3 Wolf, S., *et al.*, 'The Power of the Clan: the Influence of Human Relationships on Heart Disease' (Transaction Publishers, 1993)

4 Hong, S. and Giannakopoulos, E., 'Students' Perceptions of Life Satisfaction', *College Student Journal*, 1995, 29, 438

5 Rogers, S., 'Mothers' Work Hours and Marital Quality', *Journal of Marriage and the Family*, 1996, 58, 606

Week 6

1 Sugarman, S., 'Happiness and Population Density', Master's thesis, California State University, 1997; Coghan, C., 'An Examination of Community Action Participation' Master's thesis, University of Texas, 1989

2 Jou, Y. et al., 'Stress and Social Support in Mental and Physical Health', *Psychological Reports*, 1997, 81, 1302; Finch, J. et al., 'The Factor Structure of Received Social Support: Dimensionality and the Prediction of Depression and Life Satisfaction', *Journal of Social and Clinical Psychology*, 1997, 16, 323

3 Crist, M., 'Efficacy of Volunteerism', *Psychological Reports*, 1997, 79, 736

Week 7

1 Lundqvist, L., et al., 'Facial Expressions Are Contagious', *Journal of Psychophysiology*, 1995, 9, 203

Week 9

1 Boyce. N., 'Growing Up Too Soon', *New Scientist*, 2 August 1997, 5

Week 10

1 National Food Survey in the UK, 1995. The study confirmed that the average person is deficient in most vitamins and minerals and women are especially low in zinc which is important for female hormone problems such as PMS.

2 Schellenberg, R., 'Treatment for the Pre-menstrual Syndrome with Agnus Fruit Extract: Perspective, Randomized, Placebo Controlled Trials', *British Medical Journal*, 2001, vol. 322, 134–7

3 Sheu, S. J. et al., 'Analysis and Processing of Chinese Herbal Drugs IV: The Study of Angelicae Radix', *Planta Medica*, 1987, vol. 53, 377–8; Qi-bing, M. et al., 'Advance in the Pharmacological Studies of Radix Angelica Sinensis', *Chinese Medical Journal*, 1991, vol. 104, 776-81

4 Blake, F. et al., 'Cognitive Therapy for PMS: a Controlled Trial', *Journal of Psychosomatic Research*, 1998, vol. 45, no. 4, 307–18

5 Oleson, T. et al., 'Randomised Controlled Study of Pre-menstrual Symptoms Treated with Ear, Hand and Foot Reflexology', *Obstetrics and Gynaecology*, 1993, vol. 82, 906–11

6 Cutler, W. B. et al., 'Human Auxiliary Secretions Influence Women's Menstrual Cycles: The Role of Donor Extract from Men', *Hormones and Behavior*, 1986, vol. 20, p 463–73

Food Sources of Essential Nutrients

1 Kleijnen, J. et al., 'Vitamin B6 in the Treatment of PMS – a Review', *Journal of Obstetrics and Gynaecology*, 1990, 97, 847–52

2 Abraham, G. E., 'Nutritional Factors in PMS', *Journal of Reproductive Medicine*, 1983, 28, 446–64

3 Balch, J. F., and Balch, P. A., *Prescription for Nutritional Healing* (2nd edition, Avery Publishing Group, 1996; Murry, M. and Pizzorno, J., *Encyclopedia of Natural Medicine*, Prima Publishing, 1991

Part 3

What Your Doctor Can Offer You

1 Bancroft, J. et al., 'The Impact of Oral Contraception on the Experience of Perimenstrual Mood, Clumsiness, Food Cravings and Other Symptoms' *Journal of Psychosomatic Research*, 1993, vol. 37, 195–202

2 Carpenter, L., 'Heard the One About the Pill? It's a Killer' in Neil, K., *Balancing Hormones Naturally* (ION Press, 1994)

3 Henry, John A., (ed.), *The BMA Guide to Medicines and Drugs*, 'Hormones and Endocrine Systems' (Dorling Kindersley, 1998), p. 147

4 Theuer, Richard, 'Effect of Oral Contraceptive Agents on Vitamin and Mineral Needs: A Review', *Journal of Reproductive Medicine*, January 1972, vol. 8, no. 1

5 Kuhnz, W., et al., *Influences of High Doses of Vitamin C on the Bio Availability and the Serum Protein Binding of Levonorgestrel in Women Using a Combination Oral Contraceptive* (Elsevier Science Inc, 1995)

A-Z of PMS Symptoms and How to Beat Them

1 Snider, B. and Dieteman, D., 'Pyridoxine Therapy for Pre-menstrual Acne Flare Up', *Archives of Dermatology*, 1974, vol. 110, 130–1

2 Janiger, O. et al., 'Cross Cultural Study of PMS Symptoms', *Psychosomatics*, 1972, vol. 13, 226–35

3 Petrakis, N. L. et al. 'Cytological Abnormalities in Nipple Aspirates of Breast Fluid from Women with Severe Constipation', *Lancet*, 1981, vol. 2, no. 8257, 1203–4

4 London, R. et al., 'Mammary Dysplasia: Endocrine Parameters and Tocopherol Therapy', *Nutrition Research*, 1982, vol. 7, 243

5 Pye, J. K. *et al.*, 'Clinical Experience of Drug Treatments for Mastaglia', *Lancet*, 1985, vol. 2, 373–7; McFayden, I. J. et al., 'Cyclical Breast Pain – Some Observations and the Difficulties in Treatment', *British Journal of Clinical Practice*, 1992, vol. 46, 161–4

6 Tamborini, A. *et al.*, 'Value of Standardised Ginkgo Bilboa Extract (ECG 761) in the Management of Congestive Symptoms of PMS', *Revue Française de Gynecologie et d'Obstetrique*, 1993, vol. 88, nos 7–9, 447–57

7 Dalton, Katharina, M.D., 'Menstruation and Accidents', *British Medical Journal*, 1960, vol. 2, 1425–6

8 Kleijnen, J. *et al.*, 'Gingko Biloba', *Lancet*, 1992, vol. 340, 1136–9

9 Faccinetti, F. *et al.*, 'Magnesium Prophylaxis of Menstrual Migraine: Effects of Intracellular Magnesium', *Headache*, 1991, vol. 31, 298–304

10 Glucek, C. J. *et al.*, 'Amelioration of Severe Migraine with Omega 3 Fatty Acids: A Double Blind, Placebo Controlled Clinical Trial', *American Journal of Clinical Nutrition*, 1986, vol. 43, 710

11 Johnson, E. S. *et al.*, 'Efficacy of Feverfew as Prophylactic Treatment of Migraine', *British Medical Journal*, 1985, vol. 291, 569–73

Appendix 1

1 Bradshaw, N. D. *et al.*, 'Thyroid Hypo Function in Pre-menstrual Syndrome', *New England Journal of Medicine*, 1986, vol. 315, 1486–7

Resources

Useful Contacts

This is a list of places where you can find out more about PMS in general, your specific symptoms, and any therapies that can help you deal with PMS both physically and emotionally.

Always enclose a stamped addressed envelope when your write to an address, as many of these places are charities run by volunteers.

The Internet is also a huge source of information and support.

In addition to your doctor's advice, a PMS support group or association is a good place to start. You'll find them listed here. PMS support groups can give you advice, information and support if you need to make informed choices about your treatment options and health care.

UK

PMS

National Association for Premenstrual
Syndrome (NAPS)
41 Old Kent Road
East Peckham
Kent TN12 5AP
0870 7772177

PMS Help
PO Box 160
St Albans
Herts AL1 4UQ

Premenstrual Society (PREMSOC)
PO Box 102
London SE1 7ES

Acne

The Acne support group
PO Box 230
Hayes
Middlesex UB4 OUT
020 8561 6868

Acupuncture

British Acupuncture Council
63 Jeddo Road
London W12 9HQ
020 8735 0400

Complementary Therapies

British Complementary Medicine
Association
www.bcma.co.uk

The Natural Medicine Society
Regency House
97-107 Hagley Road
Edgbaston
Birmingham B16

Counselling

British Association for Counselling
1 Regent Place
Rugby
Warwickshire CV21 2PJ

Cognitive behavioural therapy (CBT)

Section of Psychopharmacology
Institute of Psychiatry
De Crespigny Park
London SE5 8AF

Depression

Depression Alliance
35 Westminster Bridge Road
London SE1 7JB
020 7633 9929

MIND – Mental Health Charity
15-19 Broadway
London E15 4BQ
020 8522 1728
0345 660 163

Detox – healthy lifestyle

The Breakspear Hospital
Hertfordshire House
Wood Lane
Hemel Hempstead
Herts HP2 4FD
01442 261333
Medically supervised nutritional
detox program

Environmental Air systems
Martin Wells
Sandyhill Cottage
Sandy lane
Rushmore
Tilford
Farnham
Surrey GU10 2ET

FACT – Food additives campaign team
25 Horsell Road
London N5 1XL
Healthy House
Cold Harbour
Ruscombe, Stroud
Glos GL6 6DA

The Pesticide Trust
Pesticide Exposure group of
sufferers
Eurolink centre
49 Effra Road
London SW2 1BZ
020 7274 8895

Society for Environmental Therapy
Mrs H Davidson
521 Foxhall Road
Ipswich IP3 8LW
01473 723552

Alcohol concern
275 Grey's Inn Road
London WC1X 8QF
0207 928 7377

QUIT (National Society of Non-Smokers)
102 Gloucester Place
London W1H 3DA
0207 388 5775
Smoking quitline 0800 002200

Diabetes

British Diabetic Association
10 Queen Anne Street
London W1M OBD
020 7323 1531

Eating disorders

Centre for eating disorders
020 7291 4565

Eating disorders association
Sackville Place
44 Magdalen Street
Norwich
Norfolk NR3 1JE
0160 362 1414

Overeaters anonymous
01273 624 712
Nationwide local groups

Homeopathy
British Homeopathic Association
27a Devonshire Street
London W1N 1RJ
020 7935 2163

Massage
British Federation of Massage
Practitioners
78 Meadow Street
Preston
Lancs PR1 1TS
01772 881063

Medical Herbalism
General Council and Register of
Consultant Herbalists
32 King Edward's Road
Swansea SA1 4LL
01792 655886

National Institute of Medical Herbalists
56 Longbrook Street
Exeter
Devon SX4 6AH
01392 426022
Ann Walker, PHD, MNIMH, MCPP
Senior Lecturer in Human Nutrition

School of Food Biosciences
The University of Reading
PO Box 226
Whiteknights
Reading RG6 6AP

Meditation
Transcendental Meditation Association
Free post
London SW1P 4YY
0990 143733
For TM on the NHS your doctor
will need to call the TM
communications office on 08705
143733 to request a doctor's
information pack and free video.
This will include advice on funding
for your GP.

Nutrition
British Association of Allergy,
Environmental and Nutritional
Medicine
PO Box 28
Totton
Southamptom
Hants SO40 2ZA

British Association of Nutritional
Therapists
27 Old Gloucester Street
London W1N 3XX
0870 6061284

Institute of Optimum Nutrition
Blades Court
Deodar Road
London SW15 2NU
020 8877 9993

Vegetarian Society
Parkdale
Dunham Road
Altrincham
Cheshire WA14 4QG
0161 928 0793

Vegan Society
Donald Watson House
7 Battle Road
St Leonards-on-Sea
East Sussex TN3 7AA
01424 427 393

Women's Nutritional Advisory Service
PO Box 268
Lewes
East Sussex BN7 2QN
01273 487366

Nutritional Therapists
Marilyn Glenville
Nevill Estate
Danegate
Eridge Green
Tunbridge Wells
Kent TN3 9JA
01892 750511
0906 750511

Organic Living
Food for the future foundation
51 Trevelyan
Bracknell
Berkshire RG12 8YD
01344 360033

Friends of the Earth
26-28 Underwood Street
London N1 7JQ
0808 800 1111

Green Peace
30-31 Islington Green
London N1 8XE

Organic Information
PO Box 1503
Poole
Dorset BH14 8YE
01202 715130

Organic food mail-order services
A&G Organics
01704 831 393

Farm a round
020 7627 4698

Organic direct
020 7622 3003

Sellers Organic produce
01751 472249

Simply organic
0845 1000 444
Nationwide 48-hour delivery
service

Andrews Water treatment
01704 541 578 (water distillers)

Freshwater filter company
020 8558 7495 (water filters)

Wholistic research company
01954 781074
(Can deliver juicers, water filters
and air purifiers to your door)

Chemical-free cleaning products:
The green people company Ltd
01444 401444

The Green Shop
01452 770629

Healthy house
01453 752216

Natural collection
01225 442288

Natural woman
0117 946 6649

PCOS
Verity
Grayston House
28 Charles Square
London N1 6HT
www.verity-pcos.org.uk

Supplements
Biocare Nutritional supplements
54 Northfield Road
Kings Norton
Birmingham B30 1JH
0121 433 3727

Bioforce
ww.bioforce.com
Health Plus Ltd
Dolphin House
30 Lushington Road
Eastbourne
East Sussex BN21 4LL
01323 737374

The herbalist's centre
38 New Cavendish Street
London W1M 7LH
020 7935 0405

Higher Nature Ltd
The Nutritional Centre
Burwash Common
East Sussex TN19 7LX
01435 882880

The Nutri Centre
Nutrition supplements
7 Park Crescent
London W1N 3HE
020 7436 5122

Specialist Herbal Supplies
3 Burton Villas
Hove
Sussex BN3 6BR
01273 202401

Other companies whose products are well worth trying are Solgar Vitamins (01442 890355), Lamberts healthcare (01892 552120) Viridian (01327 878050) and Quest. Ask in your local healthfood shop.

Traditional Chinese Medicine (TCM)

Register of Chinese Herbal Medicine
PO Box 400
Middlesex HA9 9NZ
020 7224 0883

Harley Street TCM healthcare
101 Bulwer Road
Leytonstone
London E11 1BU
020 8556 8843

Weight loss

Lighten Up
Pete Cohen/Judith Verity
46 Staines Road
Twickenham TW2 5AH
0845 603 3456

Vitaline Weight Control Ltd
144 Ashton Road
Manchester M34 3HR
0161 292 4919

Well Woman

Healthline
0800 55 57 77
Freephone number provided by UK department of health. Call this number to find out what treatments are available and where on the NHS.

Women's Environmental Network
87 Worship Street
London EC2A 2BE
020 7247 3327
(For information on toxins)

Women's Health
52 Featherstone Street
London EC1Y 8RT
020 7251 6580

Yoga

Yoga for health foundation
Ickwell Bury
Biggleswade
Bedforshire SG18 9EF
01767 627271

US AND CANADA

PMS

PMS Access
(Madison pharmacy associates)
PO Box 9326
429 Gammon Place
Madison W1 537I5
Toll-free number 800 558 7046
National PMS hotline
800 344 4767

The society for Menstrual cycle research
Department of Psychology
Connecticut college
New London, CT 06320
860 439 2336

Acne/skincare

American Academy of Dermatology
PO Box 4014
Schamberg, IL 60168-4014
(847) 330-0230 or (888) 462-3376

Complementary therapies

*National Clearing house for
complementary and alternative
medicine*
PB Box 8218
Silver Spring, MD 2097-8218
1-888-664-6226

Canadian Holistic Medical Association
491 Eglington Avenue West
Apt 407
Toronto
Ontario MSN 1A8
1-416-485-3071

Counselling

Concerned counselling
toll-free service within US
1-888-415-8255

Depression

Depressives anonymous
328 E 62nd Street
New York, NY 10021
(send a SAE for free information)

*National Foundation for Depressive
illness*
PO Box 2257
New York, NY 10016
(212) 268 4260

Detox

Center for environmental medicine
7510 Northforest Drive
North Charleston, SC 29420
(803) 572 1600

Environmental Protection Products, Inc
100 Canary Street
Glen Cove, NY 11542
(800) 444 3563

Friends of the Earth
530 7th Street, SE
Washington, DC 20003
(202) 543-4312

Eating Disorders
American anorexia.bulimia association
418 E 76th Street
New York, NY 10021
(212) 734 1114

Eating disorder recovery helpline
1-888-520-1700

Massage
American Massage Therapy
Association
820 Davis Street
Suite 100
Evanston, IL 60210
(312) 761 2682

Medical Herbalism
The American Herb Association
PO Box 673
Nevada City, CA 95959

Nutrition
US department of Agriculture and
nutrition information center
National Agricultural library, room
105
1031 Baltimore Ave
Beltsville, MD 20705-2351
301 504 5719

American Academy of Nutrition
College of Nutrition
3408 Sausalito
Corona del Mar, CA 92625-1638
(949) 760 6788
(Home study courses in nutrition)

American Vegan Society
501 Old Harding Highway
Malaga, NJ 08328

Food and Nutrition Information Center
National Agriculture Library
1031 Baltimore Avenue
Room 304
Beltsville, MD 20705-2351
(301) 504 5719

North American Vegetarian Society
PO Box 72
Dolgeville, NY 13329

Organic Living
You can learn about organic food
and organic living from the
following non-profit organizations:

Organic trade association
(413) 774 7511

Organic farming research foundation
(408) 426 6606

The Land Institute
(913) 823 5376

Community Alliance with family
farmers
(916) 756 8518

PCOS

Polycystic Ovarian Syndrome
Association
PB Box 80517
Portland, OR 97280

Supplements

Blessed herbs
109 Barre Plains Road
Oakham, MA 01068
(800) 489-4372

College pharmacy
833 North Tejon St
Colorado Springs
CO 80803
800 888 9358

General Nutrition center
888 462 2548
www.collegepharmacy.com

Herbal pharmacy
PO Box 116
Williams, OR 97544
(541) 846 6262

Metagenics
Nutritional Supplements
917 Calle Negocio
San Clemente, CA 92673
(714) 366 0818
(800) 692 9400

Nature's Apothecary
6350 Gunpark Dr 500
Boulder, CO 80301
(800) 999 7422

Optivite PMS supplement
800 223 1601

PMS foods Inc
LP 2701, East 11, PO Box 1099
Hutchinson, Kansas 67504-1099
800 835 5006

Schiff PMS formula
800 526 6251
www.schiffvitamins.com

Uni Key health systems
PO Box 7168
Bozeman, MT 59771
(800) 888 4353

Women's international pharmacy
5708 Monona drive
Madison, W1 53716
800 699 8144
www.womensinternational.com

Traditional Chinese Medicine

American Association of acupuncture
and chinese medicine
4101 Lake Boone Trial, Ste, 201
Raleigh, NC 27607
(919) 787 5181

Well woman

Full circle women's health
1800 30th street
Boulder
Colorado 80301 10115
303 440 7100

National Women's health Network
514 10th Street NW
Suite 400
Washington DC 20004
(202) 347 1140

OBGYN.net
The Obstetrics and Gynecology
network
5707 Lakemore
Austin, TX 50100
(512) 418 2922

AUSTRALIA

PMS

PMT Relief Clinic
Suite 6, 32 Kensington Road
Rose Park
South Australia 5067
08 364 2760

General

National Herbalists Association of
Australia
Suite 305
BST House
3 Smail Street
Broadway
New South Wales 2007
61 2 21 6437

Australian College of nutritional and
environmental medicine
13 Hilton Street
Beaumaris
VIC 3193
03 9589 6088

Australian Natural therapists (ANTA)
PO Box 308
Melrose Park
South Australia
61-8-371-3222

POSAA – *Polycystic ovary syndrome*
association of Australia
PB Box E140
Emerton
MSW 2770
612 4733 4342

Women's health advisory service
Dr Sandra Cabot
PB Box 217
Paddington
NSW 2021
02 4655 8855

Women's health statewide
64 Pennington Terrace
Nth Adelaide SA 5006
08 8267 5366

Women's information service
122 Kintore Ave
Adelaide SA 5000
08 8223 1244

HELPFUL WEBSITES

PMS
www.pms.org.uk
www.womenshealth.com
www.pop.psu.edu/smer
www.obgyn.upenn.edu/pms/pms.html
www.nlm.nih.gov/medlineplus/menstruationandpremenstrualsyndrome.html
www.project-aware.org/managing/alt/pms.html
www.4pms.com
www.goodbyepms.com
www.healthy.net/clinic/dandc/pms
www.coolpress.com (his and hers PMS calender)
www.obgyn.net

Acne and skincare
www.healthy.net/LIBRARY/BOOKS/Healthyself.acne.htm
www.m2w3.com/acne
members.tripod.com/~wildsurvival/index.html

Complementary therapies

www.bloom.com.au

www.dessertessence.com.au

www.holistichealthonline

www.internethealthlibrary.com

www.jurlique.com.au

www.thursdayplantation.com.au

Nutrition

www.patrickholford.com

www.thefooddoctor.co.uk

www.nauropathic.org

www.eatright.org

www.nutricenter.com

Organic living

www.organicfood.co.uk

www.simplyorganic.net

www.foe.co.uk/safer_chemicals (friends of the UK)

www.naturalhealtyliving.com

PCOS

www.pcossupport.org

www.posaa.asn.au

www.verity-pcos.org.uk

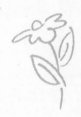

Index